For Us, the Living:

A History of U.S. Army McCloskey General Hospital, Temple, Texas

Denise Karimkhani

Dedication

This is dedicated to my parents and to the men and women of U.S. Army McCloskey General Hospital. "At a time in their lives when their days and nights should have been filled with innocent adventure, love, and the lessons of the workaday world, they were fighting in the most primitive conditions possible across the bloodied landscape of France, Belgium, Italy, Austria, and the coral islands of the Pacific. They answered the call to save the world from the two most powerful and ruthless military machines ever assembled, instruments of conquest in the hands of fascist maniacs. They faced great odds and a late start, but they did not protest. They succeeded on every front. They won the war; they saved the world. They came home to joyous and short-lived celebrations and immediately began the task of rebuilding their lives and the world they wanted."

~Tom Brokaw, *The Greatest Generation*

Preface

I was born and grew up in a world that revolved around McCloskey Veterans Hospital. Both parents, an aunt and uncle, a cousin, and countless friends and acquaintances of my family shared this common bond, and talked, gossiped, and complained about the hospital day in and day out. My parents, Aubrey Woolley and Helen Luco, met and fell in love there. My mother was a registered nurse on the orthopedics ward where my dad worked as a nursing assistant. He later went on to become a hospital fireman, guard, and policeman. Each of them completed 30 years of service at the hospital. My brother, Kyle, and I frequented the swimming pool in the summers, and it was an annual tradition to visit the hospital at Christmas to see the chapel decorated and the nativity scene on the grounds. My dad loved to talk about his experiences in World War II, and occasionally he mentioned that there had been a prisoner-of-war camp in Temple associated with the army hospital. He didn't have a lot of information, but it piqued my interest. In my job as a university librarian, I had access to print and electronic resources and spent my spare time researching and gathering information about McCloskey in hopes of one day adding to Victor Schulze's short history of the hospital.

I appreciate the research assistance of Shiloh Fulton, Jason Rushing, Jeffrey Swindoll, and Penny Worley. A special thank-you goes to Susan Claire Kimball who allowed me to use her mother's memoirs.

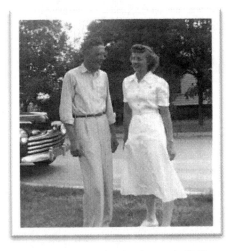

Aubrey Woolley and Helen Luco, ca. 1948

Table of Contents

Dedication
Preface

Chapter 1: A Critical Crossroads

At the beginning of the 1940s, Temple, Texas was at a crossroads. Founded as a railroad town in central Texas in 1881, Temple experienced steady growth and was well-served by a variety of businesses and cultural advantages. Three major hospitals were established in the late 19th and early 20th centuries: Santa Fe Hospital (1891), King's Daughters Hospital (1897), and Scott and White Hospital (1904).[1] In the 1920s, a welcome sign to the city declared, "Welcome to Temple, The Hospital Center of the South." [2]

Temple prospered as the largest city in Bell County until the Great Depression halted its progress. As the site of the Blackland Experiment Station, it was dominated by an agricultural economy as was most of the state. The Chamber of Commerce brochure advertised Temple as an agricultural center with a photo of "Lady Temple," a world-record-holding hen with 345 eggs in one year to her credit.[3] The State Soil Conservation Board was established in the city in May 1939, and 4,000 dirt farmers along with top soil conservationists and Governor W. Lee O'Daniel attended a state-wide meeting held in Temple. Only a few months later in July of that year, over 3,000 future farmers gathered at the Municipal Building for the organization's annual state convention. Locally, Bell County reported a decline in its 1939 cotton crop, 4,429 bales short of the previous year. In December 1939, Governor O'Daniel declared a "Cotton Christmas," to promote greater use of the fiber in retail commerce and create higher demand in the cotton markets, and thereby, do a good turn for the farmers of the state.[4]

Temple's business district was made up of a variety of enterprises, many of which had been established around the turn of the century. Ready-to-wear clothing stores like Cheeves Brothers, Roddy's, Zidell's, and Hendler's dotted the municipal landscape as did hardware, jewelry, grocery, furniture, auto, and dime stores. Temple had a dozen churches, several movie theaters, and its own radio station, KTEM Radio. Temple Junior

College boasted that it was on solid financial footing, with 1938-1939 being one of its most successful years, and the coming year promising to be even brighter.[5]

At the national level, President Franklin D. Roosevelt declared a limited national emergency in September 1939 and made it clear that he intended to prepare the U.S. for war by "strengthening of the national defense within the limits of the peacetime authorizations." [6] The following January, Roosevelt asked Congress for a national defense appropriation of 1.8 billion dollars and stated that he would like to see the United States "geared up to the ability to turn out at least 50,000 planes a year." He made a request for 1 billion dollars to procure the essential equipment for a larger and thoroughly rounded-out Army, to replace or modernize Army or Navy equipment, to increase production facilities for everything needed for the Army or Navy, and to speed up to a 24-hour basis all Army and Navy contracts.[7]

Following the decade of the Great Depression, there was a surge in patriotism, fueled by President Roosevelt who hoped to invigorate the American people and restore economic health to the country. It was sparked in 1940 with congressional passage of a joint resolution, signed by the president, declaring the third Sunday in May "I Am an American Day." Local cities and towns were encouraged to participate in any way they saw fit, celebrating those who had achieved citizenship and encouraging civic responsibility and opportunity. American citizens were acutely aware of events in Europe as their radios, newspapers, and even movies were full of war news, but many still turned a deaf ear. The country was divided among isolationists who promoted "America First" and those who believed the United States would soon be drawn into the war. Public opinion about entering World War II gradually shifted over time. However, when France fell to Germany in June 1940 and Japan moved to occupy Indo-China, views favoring isolationism continued to hold strong with 61 percent saying the United States should keep out of the conflict.[8]

By mid-1940, ordinary people began to feel the effects of the war in Europe on their daily lives. July 1st saw an increase in individual income tax rates and the imposition of defense taxes on products like beer, liquor, cigarettes, radios, matches, gasoline, playing cards, and theater tickets to raise funds for national defense and aid to Britain. Cotton prices declined with rationing abroad and loss of markets in Nazi-dominated countries. Reality hit home when men between the ages of 21 and 35 were required to register for the draft. *The Waco News-Tribune* reported that 11,057 men registered in McLennan County, and *The Bartlett Tribune* showed counts of 200 registrants in Williamson County and 173 in Bell County. During the summer and fall months, Americans listened to Edward R. Murrow's sobering broadcasts of the London blitz. Spirits brightened at the end of the year when the Temple Wildcats football team won a place in the state playoffs. Football fever gripped Bell County as the team faced the Amarillo Sandies for the state title on December 28, 1940. Most stores were closed, realizing the futility of doing business that day with the majority of the populous attending the game at the Cotton Bowl in Dallas. War, the peacetime draft, and the re-election of F.D.R. dominated 1940.

The year 1941 dawned with Adolf Hitler proclaiming that "1941 will bring the greatest completion of victory in our history. Armed as never before, we stand at the door of the New Year." [9] In contrast, President Roosevelt's State of the Union address on January 6 centered on the four freedoms: freedom of speech and religion and freedom from want and fear. By continuing to provide aid to its closest ally and increasing the production of war industries, the president argued that the United States was fighting for these universal freedoms, not only for Great Britain but for all people. Despite the dire pronouncements from politicians, Temple and the nation looked forward to the new year with a sense of optimism. A banner headline in the New Year's Day edition of *The Austin American-Statesman* announced, "Greatest U.S. Boom Due in 1941." The *Temple Daily Telegram* made a similar prediction with its headline "New

U.S. Production Peak Is Due in 1941." [10] Merchants hoped for a new year that would exceed the previous year. Based on figures from 1940, Temple businesses showed gains of from two to 23 percent. Strong Christmas sales helped some firms offset declines in the previous months. The remodeled, air-conditioned The Famous, "Temple's greatest women's store," reopened in 1940 at 13 South Main. [11] The Farmer's State Bank in Temple told of its own financial prosperity with deposits totaling an amount two hundred times greater than when it opened thirty years before. [12] It was reported that new home construction had been on the upswing since the spring of 1940.

American citizens were soon called upon to aid the war effort in new ways. In February, a "Bundles for Britain" drive kicked off to collect blankets, garments, shoes, purses, and hats for needy Britons. The first day's campaign collected more than 1,500 assorted items from Temple contributors. [13] In March 1941, Congress approved Lend-Lease aid for Britain with the idea that it was in the best interest of the United States to come to the aid of its ally whether it could pay or not. Defense savings bonds and postal saving stamps went on sale at post offices and banks nationwide May 1, 1941. A defense bond, purchased for $18.75, would be worth $25 in ten years. A limit of $5,000 was set on the amount of bonds to be bought by any one person in one year. Temple's postmaster, Nathan Roberson, sold the first defense stamps in the city to Charles L. Walker III, the young son of Mr. and Mrs. C. L. Walker, Jr. Mayor H. B. Mason bought the first bond. By the end of the first day, $8,931.23 in bonds and $279.65 in stamps were sold. [14]

The Lions' Clubs in many Texas cities and towns took the lead in collecting scrap iron for Britain's defense. Ed H. Barnes was county chairman. In Belton, Boy Scouts canvassed the town to round up scrap iron, even collecting an automobile. The Rotary Club gave cash prizes to the Scout troops bringing the most iron to add to the pile on the courthouse square. [15] A similar drive took place in Temple under the leadership of the Lions' Club. Temple's standpipe, a familiar landmark in the city located at Central Avenue and 13th Street, was torn down for scrap. The all-iron standpipe weighed 50 tons. The iron was expected to find its way into making guns and shells for Great Britain.[16] Before long, citizens were asked to contribute to the aluminum-for-defense fund for Britain and America. The national goal was 15,000,000 pounds which meant that every family needed to donate five-eighths to three-quarters of a pound of aluminum for a successful drive.[17] Temple's "March of Pans" campaign was organized by the American Legion Auxiliary, and a large group of women gathered on July 22 on the grounds of the Municipal Building to decorate the "pan pen" with red, white, and blue bunting and American flags.[18] "Pans for Planes" slips were inserted into bread wrappers as reminders, and local milk distributors did their part by collecting metal for the drive. Dr. W. A. Chernosky, a local physician, donated the section of a wing from a World War I plane.[19] By the end of the drive, three tons of aluminum were collected in Bell County, more than enough to build a fighter plane.[20]

Throughout the year, various patriotic events took place in town. KTEM broadcast a new 15-minute radio series called "Patriotism, Defense, and Brotherhood" featuring local high school students exchanging views, comments, and school news.[21] In May, Temple churches devoted a Sunday to special sermons for "I Am an American Day." To give added impetus to the Air Corps enlistment drive, Mayor Mason proclaimed August 18-23 as "Temple Keep 'Em Flying Week" to encourage individuals and civic organizations to lend their help in enlisting men for a Temple air corps unit.[22]

The summer of 1941 was characterized by Americans searching for escape from war talk by pursuing pleasurable pastimes such as movies, music, dancing, and sports. Joe DiMaggio's hitting streak drew more national attention than world events. In an August 19 press conference, President Roosevelt expressed his frustration by quoting Abraham Lincoln, "The fact is the people have not yet made up their minds that we are at war... They have not buckled down to the determination to fight this war through; for they have got the idea into their heads that we are going to get out of this fix

12

somehow by strategy."[23] Undeterred, many Americans headed for their favorite vacation destinations on Labor Day weekend for one last hurrah.

As the end of the year neared, the Temple's Christmas parade took place on the first Monday in December with eight floats, two bands, hundreds of schoolchildren in the procession, and more than 8,000 excited parade-goers lining the streets.[24] The newspaper billed the event as "the largest Christmas party and parade in the city's history." The parade seemed like a dream when one week later the Japanese bombed Pearl Harbor, ending the great debate. Finally, the country was united as the United States declared war on Japan on December 8, and on Germany on December 11. Hundreds of Bell County youth enlisted in the armed forces.

It was unfortunate but characteristic of many towns during the Great Depression that in the ten years from 1930 to 1940, Temple experienced a population decline of one person from 15,345 to 15,344.[25] This lack of growth did not escape the notice of certain area businessmen, most notably Frank W. Mayborn. As the business manager of his family-owned newspaper, the *Temple Daily Telegram*, Mayborn was keenly aware of the gathering storm in Europe and its ramifications for the United States. In the president's announcements, Mayborn foresaw the accelerated defense preparations as an opportunity for Temple and Central Texas, but he knew that he had to strike while the iron was hot. Bringing businesses and industries to Temple was the key to its survival, and there was sure to be competition from other similar cities.

Civic activism was nothing new to Mayborn who in 1939 was elected the first president of the newly created Temple Chamber of Commerce and Board of Development. An important committee of the Chamber was the Industrial Committee, tasked with bringing industry to the area. Following his tenure as president, Mayborn himself became the chairman of the Industrial Committee along with two bank presidents, the head of Scott and White Hospital, and other local businessmen. The members of the committee were W. Guy Draper, J. E.

Woods, Dr. A. C. Scott, Jr., Hill Gresham, J. E. Johnson, T. J. Cloud, Frank Jones, and Frank Matush.

His early attempts at securing a magnesium plant for the area failed but was a good learning experience. [26] Mayborn was not one to quit, and in 1940, he along with an impromptu committee, headed to Texarkana with feasibility studies touting the amenities of Central Texas in hopes of securing an army camp located in Bell County. The meeting with Senator Morris Sheppard proved fruitless as did successive efforts on the part of the Industrial Committee. [27] At every opportunity, Mayborn promoted Bell County to officials and influential friends in Washington, D.C. In the summer of 1941, rumors circulated that the War Department was seeking a minimum of 20,000 rural acres for the site of a major army base. [28] Mayborn and his committee, now called the Defense Projects Committee or War Projects Committee, quickly applied for the army base as well as an Army Air Corps training unit in Temple. [29] Before the end of 1941, news came that Temple would receive $335,000 for construction of a municipal airport. [30] But it was not until January 15, 1942 that Bell County officials learned that the army base was a reality and a Tank Destroyer Tactical and Firing Center would be located in Killeen, Texas, on 109,000 acres. [31]

Temple received its share of good news on January 6, 1942, thanks to the efforts of Frank W. Mayborn. He used the city's reputation as a hospital center as well as its location and transportation facilities to his advantage.[32] The *Telegram* reported an annual influx of as many as 25,000-30,000 patients from most states and some Latin American nations to the city's four existing hospitals and pronounced Temple "The Clinical and Surgical Center of the South."[33] The previous July, Mayborn wrote a letter to the Surgeon General of the U.S. Army and Adjutant General E. S. Adams seeking another hospital for Temple, this time an army general hospital.[34] Senator Tom Connally and Congressman W. R. Poage aided his efforts, and it was Congressman Poage who delivered the news. [35] Fort Worth, Dallas, Corsicana, and Marlin also made bids for the hospital. Colonel John R. Hall of the general medical staff and Colonel W.

Lee Hart, chief medical officer for the Eighth Corps Area recommended Temple.[36]   The January 7, 1942 *Temple Daily Telegram* announced Temple's good fortune in being selected as the site of a $2.5 million army general hospital.[37]   The previous evening Frank Mayborn read the announcement before a meeting of the Chamber of Commerce. The Chamber's War Projects Committee had been successful "beyond its wildest dreams" in bringing McCloskey General Hospital and the Army Air Field to Temple, Camp Hood to Bell and Coryell counties, and the Bluebonnet Ordnance Bomb Loading Plant to McGregor.[38] Little did the citizens of Temple realize the monumental changes that would soon come to the once small farming community in Central Texas

Chapter 2: The Wounds of War

By the time France fell in 1940, many in the United States Congress as well as the president were uneasy about the size of the U. S. peacetime force. Despite the country's neutrality, President Roosevelt called on the nation to prepare for war in addition to the production of weapons and equipment. In June, he announced that he would recommend a program of universal compulsory government service for American youth.[39] The Selective Training and Service Act of 1940 was signed into law in September, making it the first peacetime conscription law in the history of the United States.[40] The rapid buildup of troops took place in the following manner:

> A national lottery was held on October 1, 1940, to establish the order of call. On November 8, 1940, Roosevelt ordered that 800,000 men be selected and inducted by July 1, 1941. The prescribed period of active service was one year, to be followed by ten years in the reserves. On June 28, 1941, the President ordered that, during FY 1942, an additional 900,000 men would be "selected and inducted. [41]

Stephen Ambrose wrote in his history of D-Day that as a result of selective service, the average draftee was "brighter, healthier, and better educated than the average American." [42] Equipped with top-notch manpower, new weapons, and advances in combat techniques, American G.I. 's changed the ways enemies were engaged. In turn, a new way of caring for troops in combat became the focus of the wartime medical establishment.

The Medical Department of the Army, administered by the Surgeon General of the U.S. Army, was responsible for the selection and admission of healthy individuals to the service and the health maintenance of every soldier. As early as 1934, the

Surgeon General, dismayed at the state of army hospitals, sought funding from Congress, but received little more than required to maintain existing facilities. With the expansion of the armed forces, the existing hospitals would not meet the need, and the peacetime army had only 1,200 doctors. In 1939 when the president proclaimed a limited national emergency, the Medical Department was operating five general hospitals in the continental United States (Walter Reed at Washington, D.C.; Army and Navy at Hot Springs, AR.; Fitzsimons at Denver, CO.; Letterman at San Francisco, CA.; and William Beaumont at El Paso, TX.) and 119 station hospitals.[43] Station hospitals, named for the army post on which they were located, provided general care for minor ailments. General hospitals, named after deceased medical officers, were designed to provide patients with complex medical and surgical care and were under the authority and supervision of the Surgeon General of the U.S. Army. The standards for admittance to a general hospital were:

> those needing specialized treatment of the
> types for which general hospitals had been
> designated; those who would be hospitalized
> for ninety days or more; those upon whom
> elective surgery of a formidable type
> would be performed; those with specific
> types of fractures; and, with one exception,
> those evacuated from overseas theaters. [44]

Both station and general hospitals were called "named hospitals." [45]

On September 25, 1940, construction of ten new domestic general hospitals was approved. [46] In planning hospital location and construction, a variety of factors were considered: level and well-drained terrain, accessibility of transportation such as highways and railroads, water supply and utility connections, available labor, housing and commodity markets, and room for future expansion. In addition, there was a policy of locating general hospitals in areas near large training

17

camps in order to simplify the transfer of patients from station to general hospitals. Attempting to influence War Department decision-making, many local communities made attractive offers of land and utilities. In one instance, six cities offered valuable incentives when it became known that a general hospital was planned for the Fort Worth-Waco (Texas) area. Based on advice from his representatives and that of the Chief of Engineers, the Surgeon General of the U.S. Army selected the site that seemed best suited for hospital purposes. Often United States senators and representatives attempted to influence the selection of certain locations. Early in 1942, Office of the Army G-4 (Logistics) ordered all new general hospitals to be located mostly inland on a line running from Spokane to Phoenix to El Paso to Temple (Texas) to Atlanta to Cleveland, away from the coasts as a safety measure.[47] This restrictive policy created problems for distribution of patients returning from overseas theaters, and it was later abrogated. Of the 51 general hospitals authorized, acquired, or constructed between the beginning and end of the war, 28 were outside the prescribed area, 4 were on its edge and 19 were within it. Of the 28 outside the area, 9 were in the populous northeastern section of the country and 7 were in the Pacific Coast area.[48]

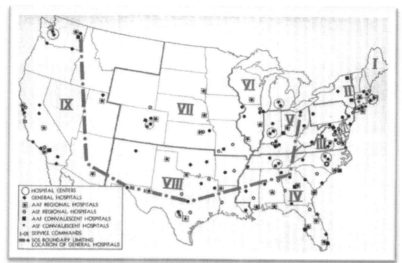

Location of General, Convalescent, and Regional Hospitals in the Zone of Interior during WW2. The Roman figures designate the 9 Service Commands. SOURCE: WW2 US Medical Research Centre, https://www.med-dept.com/articles/ww2-military-hospitals-zone-of-interior/

For new hospital buildings, the War Department utilized one-story frame construction called "cantonment-type" made of wood frame until lumber shortages set in. Building plans from 1935 prepared by the Quartermaster General in collaboration with the Surgeon General's Hospital Construction and Repair Subdivision were employed because their versatility allowed various combinations of buildings ranging in size from 25 to 2,000 beds.[49] Most buildings were a standard size and separated by 50-100 feet between for fire safety. This placement led to hospital installations that covered large areas: it was not unusual for a 500-bed hospital to spread over twenty acres. Problems and complaints surfaced as the construction got underway, and plans were found to be defective and deficient. Early in 1941, the complaints became more widespread, and by summer, work started on developing a new type of hospital. Two-story buildings with exterior walls of masonry and interiors of slow-burning materials allowed for more compact arrangement.[50] On August 6, 1941, redesigned plans authorizing construction of two-story, semi-permanent, fire-resistant plants for all future hospitals were approved.[51]

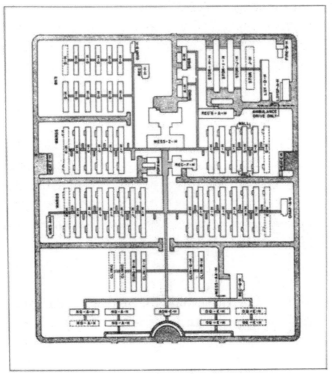

PLAN FOR TYPE A HOSPITAL

The template was referred to as a "Type A" hospital to distinguish it from earlier designs, and it featured a main administration building, compact rows of buildings organized according to use with wards for psychiatric patients isolated at the rear of the campus, medical services located near the middle, and nurses' and doctors' quarters near a public road.[52] The building schedule for Type-A hospitals included the number of buildings required per number of beds. A hospital with 1,515 beds would have an administration building, animal house, medical detachment administration and unit stores, ten medical detachment barracks, a chapel, dental and E.N.T. clinic, laboratory and professional services clinic, X-ray, gastrointestinal and physiotherapy clinic, a fire station, guard

20

house, guest house, heating plant, laundry, laundry steam plant, enlisted patients and medical detachment mess, officers' and nurses' mess, three nurses' quarters, two officers' quarters, post office, post exchange, medical detachment recreation, patients' recreation, receiving and evacuation building, shops and garage, hospital shop and morgue, medical storehouse and offices, surgery clinic, six combination wards, three detention wards, and fifteen standard wards.[53]

By the time the final drawings were completed and put into general use, the United States entered the war. In December 1941, the army had a total of about 74,250 beds in about 200 station hospitals and 14 general hospitals stateside.[54] During the next eighteen months, construction started on additional hospitals to house more than triple the number provided during the period of mobilization. In his annual report for 1942, the Surgeon General stated, "New hospital construction during the year has been for the most part of the authorized cantonment type."[55]

Fully staffing general hospitals with all the needed medical and surgical specialists was impossible because of wartime shortages. It was for this reason that army hospitals received designations as centers of special services such as amputations, chest surgery, maxillofacial and plastic surgery, ophthalmic surgery, vascular surgery, neurosurgery, and treatment of the deaf and blind. Five amputation centers were designated in March 1943, among them McCloskey General Hospital.[56] The following hospitals were designated as Amputation Centers: Bushnell General Hospital, Lawson General Hospital, Percy Jones General Hospital, Walter Reed General Hospital, and McCloskey General Hospital. In May 1943, the U.S. Army Surgeon General, Major General James C. Magee, held a conference in Washington, D.C. for the purpose of "coordinating and standardizing the treatment and fitting of amputees."[57] Information and directives were published relative to surgical principles and a uniform system of prosthesis-fitting was adopted. [58]

Like other medical specialties during World War II, physical therapy faced significant problems when the president proclaimed a limited national emergency in 1939. The most serious problem was a shortage of professional personnel. The army wanted one physical therapist per 100 beds in hospitals in the Zone of Interior. [59] In 1941, a War Emergency Training Course at Walter Reed General Hospital, under the supervision of Emma Vogel, was initiated to train civilians to be physical therapists. [60] Initially, ten students were authorized, and the 26 weeks of didactic instruction included "intensive study in anatomy, physiology, pathology, kinesiology, and allied subjects and thorough study and practice in the techniques of the various physical therapeutic procedures and their application to the specialized fields of military medicine." [61] Special emphasis was placed on the treatment of patients with combat injuries. Classroom study was followed by six months of practice at a military hospital. The graduates were called physiotherapy aides instead of reconstruction aides as they had been called during World War I. Unfortunately, one course did not meet the need for personnel so four additional courses were added at other general hospitals.

Another plan to meet the procurement requirements for physical therapists was in the works. The idea was to offer Army physical therapy courses to qualified enlisted women. The plan offered opportunities for advancement since the women would be eligible to apply for commissions as second lieutenants upon completion of the course. The institutions selected to provide training under the War Department contract were Stanford University, the University of Wisconsin, and the D. T. Watson School of Physiotherapy.[62] In December 1943, the Secretary of War authorized the direct recruitment of women qualified for the Women's Army Corps for the specific purpose of attending physical therapy training courses, with the assurance of a commission as a physical therapist upon satisfactory completion of the course if otherwise qualified. This proved to be a productive program evidenced by the fact that the number of women recruited for this specific program comprised more than half of the total military enrollment in these courses.[63]

The situation was worse for recruiting and training occupational therapists. When the United States entered the war in December 1941, there were eight qualified occupational therapists and four occupational therapy assistants on duty in five Army hospitals.[64] The Army experienced difficulties recruiting occupational therapists primarily because the Surgeon General of the U.S. Army, Major General James C. Magee, decided to appoint occupational therapists as civilian employees of the Medical Department instead of giving them a commission in the army. Another war emergency training course was implemented for occupational therapists as had been done for physical therapists. Qualified applicants were required to possess (1) a Bachelor of Science or Bachelor of Arts degree, with a major in arts and crafts; industrial art, with teacher training experience; home economics, including manual skills; or fine or applied arts, including manual skills; and (2) basic psychology. The only additional requirements of candidates accepted for this training were that they be citizens of the United States and between the ages of 21 and 35. [65] Students spent four months of classroom study on medical subjects and the theory and application of occupational therapy followed by eight months of clinical practice as apprentices in designated Army general hospitals. On February 22, 1945, the Surgeon General requested permission to increase from 600 to 700 the total number of students to be trained in the War Emergency Course.[66] In June 1945, four occupational therapists graduated from McCloskey in the first class of its kind in the United States under the War Emergency program. General Bethea presented diplomas in red leatherette frames to Miss June Hollis (Cameron, TX.), Miss Nancy Preece (San Antonio, TX.), Miss Anna Louise Master (Houston & Dallas, TX.), and Miss Marsella Bundtrock of Wyoming. Lieutenant D. T. Pierce, chief of occupational therapy, presented their caps. Miss Edna Vehlow, senior therapist, recited a resume of each therapist's training.

Jack Piarson of Joplin, Missouri, a McCloskey patient, sang "Water Boy."[67]

As a vital part of the care team, dietitians were in demand but also in short supply. A model curriculum had been implemented at Walter Reed General Hospital in 1922. By August 1942, 211 dietitians had graduated from the student training course, but an accelerated program was needed to meet the needs of World War II. At different times during the war, enlisted members of the Women's Army Corps with backgrounds in home economics expressed an interest in the Army student dietitian training course. On March 6, 1945, enlisted women were permitted for the first time to apply for assignment to the six-month apprentice training course. The Surgeon General's Office authorized the establishment of the first training course for enlisted members of the Women's Army Corps at McCloskey General Hospital with ten apprentices in each class. Five applicants were accepted, and upon completing the course, they were commissioned as Medical Department dietitians.[68] The course began on June 15, 1945 and was discontinued on January 1, 1946.

Dietitians planned hospital menus designed to satisfy the food habits of the majority with consideration given to many other factors such as climate, season, availability and cost of foods, adequacy of equipment, and skills of the mess personnel. The Office of the Quartermaster General issued a monthly master menu as a guide for hospitals. [69] Hospitals had menu planning boards composed of the mess officer, the assistant mess officer, the director of supply, and the head dietitian that met regularly to discuss issues in menu planning. The dietitian furnished standardized recipes and instructions to cooks to ensure high-quality, uniform products within the ration allowance, and checked on proper use of leftovers, meat scraps, fat, etc., to avoid unnecessary food loss. The dietitian made rounds of the wards during mealtime to assess the quality of the food and the appearance of the food trays. Direct contact with patients enabled her to get feedback on their likes and dislikes.

Two types of food service were utilized in army hospitals to accommodate different types of patients—ward and mess hall:

Mess service included cafeteria, family style, and waiter. Generally, waiter service was given to orthopedic patients, wheelchair patients, such as paraplegics, and to officer personnel. Adjustments were made in the height of tables to accommodate the wheelchairs. The change of surroundings from the ward environment improved the morale of these patients as well as those patients on therapeutic diets, who were served in the dining hall.[70]

The dietitian and army nurse worked closely, and it was the nurse who was responsible for preparation and service of trays in ward diet kitchens. Ward food service presented some difficulties, primarily the inability to keep food hot or cold and the availability of amenities such as condiments.

A nursing shortage was another problem faced not only by the army but the nation when the United States entered the war. When Pearl Harbor was bombed, there were fewer than 7,000 nurses in the Army Nurse Corps.[71] The American Red Cross was tasked with recruiting nurses for both the Army and Navy Nurse Corps. To increase the nurse power in the United States, Congress passed the Bolton Act (P.L. 74) in 1943 to prepare and train nurses more rapidly. The Bolton Act provided federal funds to maintain all students who joined the U.S. Cadet Nurse Corps and subsidized nursing schools that would provide accelerated training in a two-and-a-half-year program. Tuition, fees, books, and living expenses were provided as well as a monthly stipend. Graduates of the program promised to engage in military or civilian nursing for the duration of the war. They were also eligible to become registered nurses. By 1943, there were 100,486 student nurses enrolled nationwide.[72]

On the local front in Temple, the training programs at Scott and White Hospital and King's Daughters Hospital made efforts to train more nurses by tripling their admissions numbers.[73] By June 1944, McCloskey was home to 16 senior cadet nurses, and hundreds more arrived in the next four years. In 1945, 265 cadet nurses reported for duty during the year; 141 completed their training; and 104 were present for duty by the end of the year.[74] The cadets in the first group had between two to four and a half months of instruction remaining before graduation. Captain Mildred V. Lucka, director of the cadet nursing program at the hospital said,

> Both patients and duty personnel have been anxious for their coming. Due to our extreme shortage of nurses, we shall be most appreciative of the help the cadets will give us, and being stationed here will be an unusual opportunity for them since they will find many disease conditions they have never seen before. We know these nurses are vitally interested in the type of
> work here at McCloskey as coming to an
> Army hospital is purely voluntary.[75]

The Christmas menu of December 1944 included an employee roster and listed 126 women who were in the Army Nurse Corps, 31 senior cadet nurses, 31 nurses' aides, and 26 American Red Cross nurses.[76] Yet in December 1944, Lieutenant Colonel Zita Callaghan, chief nurse at McCloskey, continued to warn of the grave shortage of nurses:

> The war news shows that the number of our
> wounded men is growing. Only by individual
> nursing and care, can we bring them back
> to health again. This will take a great number
> of nurses than ever before to perform the
> task of healing. We cannot afford to overlook
> this plea for American women to come to the
> side of our fighting men. [77]

26

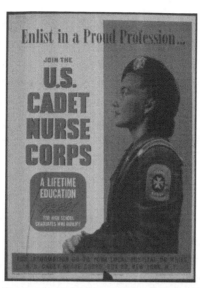

McCloskey's training program for cadet nurses was the largest of any army hospital with 110 cadet nurses per class. The cadet nurses also served rotations through Scott and White Hospital and King's Daughters Hospital. Nine cadet nurses from Methodist Hospital and Baylor University Hospital arrived at McCloskey in June 1944 for the last phase of their training. The girls were Jeffie Cannon (Jacksboro, TX.), Violet E. Goldsmith (Quitman, TX.), Melba I. Brooks (Timpson, TX.), Dorrance J. Woodridge (Austin, TX.), Doris J. Visingard (Dallas, TX.), Wanda L. Rayford (Stanton, TX.), Mary I. Rife (Pampa, TX.), Jessie M. Cannon (Dallas, TX.), and Dorothy E. Tait (Sherman, TX.). Other girls came from Mercy Hospital in New Orleans, St. Anthony Hospital in Oklahoma City, and Jefferson Davis Hospital in Houston. When asked about their impressions of McCloskey, the girls had high praise for the program, the opportunity to obtain valuable training, the friendliness and hospitality of the staff, and the new and modern equipment.

In July 1945, McCloskey graduated a Women's Army Corps class of 225. The women took four to six weeks of basic training and further specialized training at Fort Oglethorpe,

Georgia before reporting to McCloskey. At the hospital they rotated among the wards and services and attended lectures and demonstrations on ward administration. While at McCloskey, they were under the command of Captain Pearl Wood. The outstanding graduates included Private Edna Black (Houston, TX.); Private Delema Burch (Washington, IN.); Private Sylvia Wineberger (Cleveland Heights, OH.); and Private Regina Anderson (Ormsby, PA.).

Prior to World War II, there had been no special training programs in the army for psychiatric nurses. There were unsuccessful attempts to establish formal courses in some army hospitals. In the fall of 1944, the service commands were encouraged to establish their own schools for neuropsychiatric nursing. The Eighth Service Command established its course at McCloskey General Hospital on October 20, 1944. Five courses of three months' duration were offered, graduating a total of 71 students. The course provided 32 hours of didactic instruction in psychiatry, 10 hours in military psychiatric administration, 4 hours on liaison with special services, and 62 hours in psychiatric nursing. The course was given under the direction of Lieutenant Colonel Guy C. Randall, MC, chief of the neuropsychiatric service, and Captain Madeline Weiss, ANC.[78]

Nurses' aides were part of the McCloskey team, and *The Austin American-Statesman* of May 21, 1944, told a delightful story of eight girls in pinafores who came to the hospital from various parts of the country to do their patriotic duty. [79] Seven aides trained in Houston, and the eighth was from Dallas. They all originally volunteered to serve at McCloskey as Red Cross aides without pay. However, before they arrived, the government gave them a civil service rating, allowing them to be paid $62.08 after all deductions, including war bonds, were made. Room, board and laundry were also provided, and they were housed and fed with the regular army nurses. Not knowing where to go upon arrival, the girls saw an ambulance at the train station and persuaded the driver to take them to General Bethea at the hospital. One girl said, "The driver's eyes like to have popped out. Of course, the general's secretary sent us to

Lieutenant Colonel Zita Callaghan, chief nurse." Then the driver proceeded to take them to the wrong living quarters which involved much loading and unloading of luggage. The aides received uniforms of the Red Cross volunteer nurses' aide corps and were required to pay for six uniforms which consisted of a pinafore, blouse, cap, and stockings. Cost of the pinafores was $1.80, the blouses, $1.56, and caps, 50 cents each. Stockings were the most expensive items and wore out quickly. The girls worked eight-hour shifts, six days a week. Their duties included giving baths, taking temperatures, bandaging wounds, and a myriad of other tasks needed in hospital wards, such as manicures, pedicures, shampoos, and shaves. Several of the girls gave up jobs in the private sector to enter the army service. Miss Wilma Rogers left Houston Power & Light to work in the neurosurgery ward; Miss Lorene Medford, working for the Lykes Steamship Lines, sacrificed her job to serve in the plastic surgery ward; Mrs. Monte Stuckey, the wife of a Pasadena judge, took the Red Cross nursing course in hopes that she might be called on to help; Miss Joy Lowe, formerly employed at Shell Oil Company and assigned to the orthopedic ward, found satisfaction in doing things that injured arms and legs couldn't do for themselves; Miss Marion Enholm previously worked at the ferry command in Dallas and transferred to McCloskey where she reportedly gained fifteen pounds after arriving; Miss Evelyn Simmons was assigned to the surgical ward and expressed her excitement at seeing a patient move his hand or leg for the first time after being injured; and Miss Anna Munger told of going to parties and weddings in the wards, listening to patients' love stories and troubles, and her pure enjoyment of work at the hospital as she waited for her fiancé, a Navy doctor stationed somewhere in the Pacific.

Chapter 3: A Hope Realized

When Representative Poage wired the highly anticipated details of the army hospital to officials in Temple, they included location, numbers of buildings and employees, and possible future expansion. The text of the telegram read:

> Army has made me announcement and no
> order has yet been issued, but I have definite
> information indicating Temple has been selected
> as site for general base hospital. I have been in
> close contact with army officials. Hospital
> will be 1,500-bed unit with plans already
> drawn to double size if needed. First
> unit will employ 80 doctors, 170 nurses, and
> 700 enlisted men in addition to civilian
> personnel. Will serve all Texas and probably west
> coast. Estimated cost of first unit $2,500,000.
> Occupancy expected within five months. Bids
> will be advertised for 100 wooden buildings
> and at the same time an alternative bid will
> be asked for 50-two-story permanent
> fireproof buildings. I am strongly urging use
> of permanent fireproof construction and
> feel sure this will be used unless bids develop
> too great a difference is cost. This makes
> it certain Temple will always remain the
> hospital center of the South. Congratulations.[80]

The hospital's designation was authorized on January 6, and on January 21, the Secretary of War directed the immediate acquisition of land. The site chosen by the War Department was 215 acres at the south edge of the city between Highway 36 and the Katy Railroad tracks, extending from Avenue O on the north to the Katy underpass on the south. The Chamber of Commerce was responsible for the acquisition of land for the government, and by February 10 had obtained deeds on 160 of the 215 acres. T. J. Cloud noted that the "options all were obtained at reasonable prices and the property owners were showing commendable spirit of cooperation and patriotism." During the preliminary investigation of the hospital's location, the Temple City Commission voted to order a bond election to finance the land in the event of Temple's selection. As soon as official word came, an election was set for February 16, 1942, in which citizens would vote to approve or disapprove the following proposals: $22,500 in matching funds for expanded park and recreation facilities; $12,500 for a new police station and jail; and $50,000 to purchase the land for the army hospital.[81] The bond issue passed overwhelmingly, and the hospital was scheduled to be completed by September 15, 1942. Temple was supported in the bond issue by Tom DuBose of Belton who purchased $62,000 in bonds from the city at 2.25 percent interest.[82] Preparing for the challenges ahead, Temple's mayor H. B. Mason appointed a Temple Executive Defense Council with members Tucker Wyche, C. C. Bradshaw, R. L. St. John, O. F. Gober, George Hoherd, Frank Boulding, A. E. Taylor, and W. R. Brown.[83]

Joseph Roman Pelich was the supervising architect of the army hospital in joint venture with Wiley G. Clarkson, Preston M. Geren, Sr., and Joe Rady.[84] The distinguished, award-winning team was responsible for designing numerous hospitals, airfields, and other defense facilities in Texas. Captain Gordon P. Larson of the Engineer Corps supervised the actual construction until his transfer to Denver. On March 10, Lieutenant Donald W. Waterman was appointed area engineer in charge of the job. Grading and dirt work crews with Bell & Braden of Amarillo began excavation work on March 7, planning to move 10,000 cubic yards of earth per day for a total of 250,000 cubic yards.[85] The *Temple Daily Telegram* reported that crowds of spectators gathered to watch crews clear, excavate, and prepare the site. Excavated dirt was used to fill in gullies running north and south at the site. Bell & Braden also laid the gravel base for roads and built concrete drainage pipes. Building contractors' bids were due March 30 to the Eighth Corps Area Engineer's office. Construction of McCloskey General Hospital was awarded to the American Construction Company of Houston and commenced on April 16, 1942, with an average of 800 men employed daily, peaking at 2,200 at one time.[86] By the end of May, thirty-three buildings were under construction.[87]

The hospital was not an ordinary cantonment hospital. It was constructed of dull red Texas brick on the outside backed with hollow tile and with plaster on the inside.[88] Flooring was provided by Joe Stanley Flooring of Houston; electrical installation by Allan Cooke Electric of Houston; boiler foundations and installation by Mechanical Equipment of Houston and J. W. Mundy Construction of El Paso; cold storage rooms by Alfred Reed Company of Austin; and overhead electrical by Ashe Electric of Fort Worth.[89] The city of Temple supplied a water main and sewer line at a cost of $10,000. Using the city's storage tanks with a capacity of 500,000 gallons of water each, lines connected with the hospital on Avenue P, on Eighth Street, and on First, Second, and Eighth Streets.

Other important construction projects were taking place in town. The Surgeon General recommended and approved the construction of a temporary Army Hospital Training Center across the highway from the McCloskey reservation. The center was designed to house 1,000 staff members to oversee the training of personnel who would be sent to field hospitals in combat zones. Transportation resources needed improvement to speed up hospital construction and to convey patients. Widening South First Street from downtown was of utmost importance. Santa Fe Railroad announced that it would build a spur line on Tenth Street from the depot to the hospital to accommodate hospital trains.[90] In July 1942, the U.S. Army Air Forces acquired land west of Temple adjacent to Highway 36 and started construction of the Temple Army Air Field which was a substation of Waco Army Air Field and intended to be temporary in nature.[91] By the end of the year, the Southwestern Transit Company installed a new city bus line with a special McCloskey route to aid those having business at the hospital.

Buses arrived every hour on the hour, and the fare for a single passenger was seven cents.

Temple soon became a city of unprecedented activity. City fathers prepared for the arrival of thousands of soldiers in town by enhancing recreational facilities and programs. The U.S.O. was granted use of the Y.M.C.A. building which had its own swimming pool, dance hall, badminton courts, bowling alley, and reading room.[92] On weekends, professional wrestling was featured at the Municipal Auditorium with part of the proceeds going to the city recreation fund.

The simultaneous building of Camp Hood and the army hospital in Temple placed a strain on the labor force and housing situation in Bell County. The headquarters for the army camp began operations in Temple on February 17, 1942, with a staff of thirty officers and several civilian employees.[93] Belton opened an employment office to enlist and process 12-15,000 construction workers for the projects.[94] Early on, some Temple citizens expressed concern over the rapid expansion of the city and feared neglect of the agricultural industries that had been the mainstays of the county's economy. Hill C. Gresham, vice-chairman of the Temple Chamber of Commerce Defense Projects Committee, penned the following column for the local newspaper:

> The building of a large government airport here
> with its attendant activity; the construction
> and operation of the army camp at Killeen which
> will house 35,000 men; the establishment
> of a general army hospital with its 80 doctors, 170
> nurses and some 800 additional personnel, provide
> the people and businessmen of Temple with a big
> topic for conversation. The prospects for
> economic benefits are greater than they have been
> for a long time. We have ceased to worry about five
> cent cotton. Now that cotton has gone to 20 cents,
> we show little concern or enthusiasm. The most
> stimulating indoor sport seems to be the contempla-

33

tion of the good business which these government projects will bring. With this good business which is expected, however, attendant problems present themselves. A few of our far-sighted citizens have been thinking about them; eventually all of us will be forced to do so. The responsibilities are many and great; the problems are taking form and must be solved early.[95]

The massive influx of soldiers, civilian employees and their families, and construction workers quickly resulted in a housing shortage and rising rents all over Bell County. It was reported in the *Belton Journal* that Belton alone needed two thousand new homes to accommodate both the military and civilian population who were crowded into garages, basements, apartments, and rooms with no relief in sight. The task of providing shelter was made more difficult by the government's war ban on building materials, and the *Journal* editorial advocated for its lifting.[96] As time went on, the housing shortage intensified, and by April, the Temple area was declared a "private housing priority locality."[97] National Housing Administrator Harry Knowlton advised that 185 houses, not to exceed $6,000 in cost, were to be built with plans approved by the War Production Board. It was expected that Temple's quota would be increased following a new survey of housing. Not less than 50% of new houses were required to be available for rent at a cost of $50 or less per month with preference being given to defense workers. Additional regulations required location of housing within walking distance of the war activity it served or within walking distance of adequate, affordable public transportation. Labor became scarcer as men working on the projects were drafted for the war. The Works Progress Administration cancelled seven projects in the Temple area to free up labor for Camp Hood and the army hospital.[98] In June 1942, the *Temple Daily Telegram* stated that although 2,000 men were employed on the hospital construction project, more bricklayers and plasterers were needed immediately.[99] The

Central City Commercial College (Four-C College) in Waco solicited students who wanted to train for defense projects in the area including the Bluebonnet Ordnance Plant in McGregor, the Waco Army Flying School, the Blackland Army Airfield in China Spring, Camp Hood in Killeen, and McCloskey Hospital in Temple.[100] Temple merchants addressed the Hearne Defense Clinic to discuss the many problems that plagued the city with the influx of construction workers and an extreme housing shortage. Hearne had been selected as the site of a large prisoner-of-war camp.

On July 2, 1942, Mrs. James A. McCloskey was notified that the army hospital was to be named for her husband, the first Regular Medical Office killed in World War II. [101] The Surgeon General wrote in part,

> In accordance with the recommendation
> submitted by me, the War Department has
> designated the new Army general hospital now
> under construction at Temple, Texas, as the
> McCloskey General Hospital, as a tribute to, and
> to do honor to, the memory of your husband. I
> would like … to express the hope that this
> recognition of and perpetuation of the name of
> your husband may help assuage your grief in
> the knowledge that his sacrifice is not unnoted by
> his colleagues still in the service, who will
> continue to carry on the fight, and by a grateful
> nation. [102]

Major James Augustus McCloskey, a native Texan, was stationed in the Philippines in 1942 and was killed on March 26 when he went to Bataan in a military command car to check on supplies. A Japanese aircraft bombed the car in which he was riding. McCloskey attempted to run but was hit by shell fragments and was dead upon arrival at hospital. He was buried in the American Military Cemetery at Fort McKinley in the Philippine Islands. In his final letter to his wife, Marian, Major

McCloskey wrote, "The going is hard, but the fight is well worth it."[103]

Temple businesses closed, and schoolchildren were released for this grand occasion in the city's history.

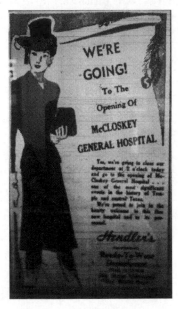

Newspaper ad for Hendler's Ready-to-Wear Department Store, Temple, Texas.
SOURCE: *Temple Daily Telegram,* November 4, 1942.

The formal opening for the first unit was November 4, 1942 at 3:00 p.m. with dedication ceremonies taking place in front of Building 1, the hospital's administration building.[104] Music was provided by the Camp Hood Band. The exercises began with formal delivery of the hospital to Colonel Bethea and the Medical Department by Area Engineer, Lieutenant Donald W. Waterman. Reverend J. B. Dobbins of Christ Episcopal Church offered the dedication prayer. Major W. H. Vaughan read a message from the Surgeon General, and Major Leslie Maurer of the U.S. Army Medical Corps and Chief of Dental Services at McCloskey delivered a eulogy in memory of his friend, James McCloskey, with whom he attended St. Mary's Academy in San Antonio.[105] Major General Richard Donovan, commanding general of the Eighth Service Command, gave an address followed by the main dedication address offered by W. R.

Poage.[106]   Government and city officials as well as family members of Major McCloskey were in attendance.   Mrs. McCloskey and her eight-year-old son, Robert, and Major McCloskey's parents, Judge and Mrs. Augustus McCloskey of San Antonio were on the platform as guests of honor.[107] Also in attendance were his aunt, sister, and brother. Prior to the ceremony, Colonel Bethea wrote to Mrs. McCloskey requesting a portrait of her husband for the dedication service. The letter, dated August 6, 1942, said,

> Dear Mrs. McCloskey, I have received a communication which Colonel Dolan wrote the Chamber of Commerce in regard to dedication exercises for this hospital. Nothing definite is planned at the present time, and as soon as we have any definite plans, I will let you know. We will certainly feel honored if you can be present for these exercises. My own opinion is that dedication exercises for military establishments in war time should be very simple and brief. We are very anxious to have a large picture of Major McCloskey to hang in a conspicuous place in our hospital; and we are very much in hopes that you can furnish us with this. I regret very much that I never had the pleasure of knowing Major McCloskey but some of my friends who knew him intimately have sung his praises to me; and we all feel that our hospital is honored by being named for him.[108]

Following the dedication exercises, the hospital was open to the public for tours. Tea for the general public was served in the Red Cross Building by the Volunteer Canteen Corps; a special tea for distinguished guests was provided in the Nurses' Quarters by invitation only. To end the day, the Gideons of Texas presented 40 Bibles, 100 Nurses' Testaments, and 1,000 Soldiers' Testaments to the hospital in the Red Cross

Building.[109] The first phase of the hospital was completed in seven months, encompassing 18.7 acres with over three miles of corridors.[110] Rumors circulated that messengers might be equipped with skates or bicycles to travel the long hallways! In his memoirs, James Bethea lauded the hospital as a beautiful institution, but "spread out too much in spite of the buildings being two-storied." [111] One newspaper reported that McCloskey "is so large that men on the north wards speak of men on the opposite wards as living 'down South.'" [112]

In September 1942, Representative W. R. Poage sent word that the size of the hospital would be doubled with a $3 million expansion with a total of 3,000 beds. Shortly after, construction began on the second phase. The original hospital plans called for duplicate buildings throughout -- two of everything -- but there was not an exact duplication of the first unit. Instead, five brick barracks for enlisted soldiers were converted into wards and sixteen new temporary barracks along with a mess hall and recreation rooms were constructed in the southeast corner of the reservation called the detachment area. The construction of the second unit of 1,500 beds had been underway since the previous September, and by June 16, 1943, McCloskey General Hospital was officially completed. The hospital took over an annex in Waco, thus providing a total of 4,600 patient beds.[113]

A year later residents of Temple and military dignitaries gathered to celebrate McCloskey's one-year anniversary. The newspaper stated, "the army's setup here [is] the most expensive in the nation." [114] A parade with all units of the hospital and the 94th General Hospital (in training) followed a one-hour concert on the quadrangle in front of the administration building. Guest of honor and speaker was Brigadier General Charles R. Glenn, Army Air Forces Training Command in Fort Worth. Two Air Medals, three Silver Stars, 26 Purple Heart awards, and 141 Good Conduct ribbons were presented.[115] Soon after, the Temple City Commission passed a city ordinance including the hospital within the city limits.[116]

Ernest V. Kunz, the manager of St. Anthony Hotel in San Antonio, commissioned Texas artist, Victor Lallier, to paint a portrait of Major McCloskey to be gifted to the hospital at its second anniversary. As the two-year anniversary of the hospital neared in the fall of 1944, General Bethea corresponded with Mrs. McCloskey regarding her husband's portrait,

> Mr. Victor Lallier, the artist who is painting the portrait of Major McCloskey, tells us that it will be ready for formal presentation on our anniversary, November 4th. Of course, we want you and your son and Mr. and Mrs. Augustus McCloskey, to be present. We are not going to have a party or open house, but we are going to present this portrait at a formal retreat ceremony at 4:30 P.M. on November 4th. Of course, we will expect all members of the McCloskey family to be our guests while here, and we have facilities for keeping you overnight if you so desire." [117]

The presentation of the portrait was the highlight of the celebration. The portrait was hung in post library no. 2.[118]

The opening of McCloskey General Hospital in 1942 marked a new era in the growth of Temple, both economically and culturally. In the beginning, the monthly payroll was expected to exceed half a million dollars. The hospital served thousands of patients as well as friends and relatives who arrived in town to visit. Temple farmers had a new lease on life with a ready-made market as they were called upon to provide chickens, eggs, milk, cream, beef, pork, and fresh produce for McCloskey. Merchants anticipated significant increases in retail business. Temple was thrilled at the prospect of its new populous made up of "citizens above average," as one columnist wrote,

They are men and women of science; they are students; they are well-educated; and they value the things which make life so worth living. Such people and their families, living in Temple, will profoundly influence the lives of each of us and our civic life. These people are above the average in mentality and in education. They know and appreciate the better things and exert a tremendous influence for good which is felt in our schools, in our churches, in our business institutions, and in our daily lives. No part of our civic enterprise is quite free from it, and every part has been improved because of it.[119]

Chapter 4: A City Within a City

The hospital was in the early stages of construction when Colonel James A. Bethea arrived in mid-June 1942. Bethea had just completed a tour as Chief of the Surgical Service at Fort Sam Houston when he was ordered to Temple to administer the new general hospital as its chief medical officer. He was 55 years old and had been in the army for over 25 years.[120] Upon his arrival, he found that he was alone except for the company of a couple of engineers. As Bethea said,

> "I didn't even have a postage stamp, much less an office or typewriter, or a nickel to spend. I borrowed money for a long-distance call from the engineer, phoned the Surgeon General's office and told him I wanted orders by wire to go to Washington. I promptly got the orders, went to Washington for a few days, and came home with authority to hire employees, buy or rent equipment, etc. I then brought up from Fort Sam Houston a group of people that had requested to come to Temple with me."[121]

Upon his return from Washington, Colonel Bethea proceeded to staff the hospital. McCloskey followed the Surgeon General's lead in developing protocols for surgical reconstruction, reconditioning and rehabilitation by bringing together multidisciplinary teams of physicians, nurses, dietitians, therapists, and prosthetists to work together on the complex injuries. For the first time, women entered professional training programs for physical therapy, occupational therapy, dietetics, and nursing to meet the needs of the newly constructed general hospitals. On the day of the hospital's dedication, medical observers expressed high hopes that Temple would be the birthplace of important medical advancements in rehabilitation of war casualties.

Two officers assigned to McCloskey were Major W. H. Vaughan and Lieutenant Orin E. Strande. [122] Vaughan was a Medical Corps officer whom Bethea appointed as his executive officer. Strande was a medical administrative officer who became the supply officer. Bethea selected Lieutenant Charley H. Freeman, an Oklahoma druggist as the adjutant, and Lieutenant John W. Cunningham as the mess officer. Registrar of McCloskey was Major I. Herbert Scheffer. Chief of the Medical Service was Major Sloan G. Stewart, and Lieutenant Foy Roberson headed the Surgical Service.[123] Major Paul G. F. Schmitt was Chief of the Laboratory Service; Captain David M. Earl was Chief of the X-Ray Service; and Major Leslie D. Maurer headed up the Dental Service.[124] Captain Zita Callaghan, Principal Chief Nurse, had spent 25 years soldiering from South Carolina to China to the Philippines prior to her arrival at McCloskey.[125] From the beginning there was an esprit de corps among the hospital staff. The motto of "Happiness, Kindness, Efficiency" seen on Colonel Bethea's desk set a pattern for morale among the doctors which carried over to the other staff and patients.

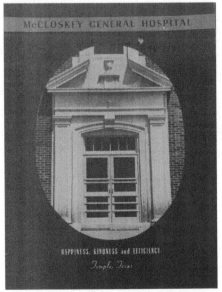

Cover of booklet, *McCloskey General Hospital: Happiness, Kindness and Efficiency, Temple, Texas*, n.d. SOURCE: Olin E. Teague Veterans' Center Medical Library Archives.

In October 1942, before the hospital was officially open, Bethea received an urgent wire asking when the hospital could receive patients. He responded that the hospital could receive patients immediately as the construction project was nearing completion. At Bethea's urging, the contractor scheduled twenty-four-hour shifts, and the enthusiastic construction workers had the hospital ready in ten days. Work was completed on October 23, 1942. McCloskey received its first patient, Private Overton Harrah, from Ansted, West Virginia, on October 20, 1942. He was admitted to Ward 16-A. Two days later ninety-seven additional patients arrived for treatment and observation.

When phase one of the hospital was complete, it consisted of 54 two-story, red brick buildings with green asphalt tile roofs, all connected by covered and heated walkways except for the service buildings and warehouses at the extreme rear of the property. The gradually sloping ramps and adjacent stairways eliminated the need for elevators. Opening-day staff at McCloskey consisted of 140 doctors, 240 nurses, 400 enlisted men, and 850 civilian employees including technicians, clerks, stenographers, janitors, gardeners, and others.[126] According to the commander, there were 65 employees per patient.[127] At the first staff assembly, Colonel Bethea directed his employees to "make McCloskey the United States Army's finest hospital." [128]

It was a monumental task to oversee such a large-scale operation, enforce regulations, and maintain practical communication. The general organization of the hospital closely paralleled that of the Eighth Service Command Headquarters and conformed to the detailed provisions of TM 8-260 (War Department Technical Manual, *Fixed Hospitals of the Medical Department (General and Station Hospitals)*), AR 40-600 (U.S. Army, *Medical Service: Medical Treatment Facilities*), and AR 40-590 (*Organization of the Surgical Service*). Beginning in October 1942, Colonel Bethea issued *The Daily Bulletin*, usually a one-to-two-page typewritten newsletter, to disseminate both official and unofficial information in the form of orders and memoranda to employees. The post newspaper, *The Caducean*, was published weekly by soldiers at the hospital and featured articles about sports, training, civilians, chaplain services, and chuckles and fun. Additional material was supplied by the Camp Newspaper Service. The Waco Annex published its own newsletter, *The Reconditioner.* The *Directory of Officers* listed officers by rank with their post assignment, home address, and home and office telephone numbers.

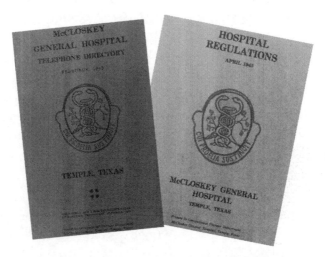

McCloskey Hospital Telephone Directory & Hospital Regulations.
SOURCE: Olin E. Teague Veterans' Center Medical Library Archives.

By the end of the war, McCloskey was a "vast geometric pattern" of 94 permanent buildings, 96 temporary buildings, a nine-hole golf course, bowling alleys, Olympic-size tile swimming pool (150' x 100'), tennis and handball courts, baseball diamonds, and a modern gymnasium, facilities that aided physical therapy as well as offered recreational opportunities for the veterans.[129] Within the hospital reservation were seven kitchens, eight mess halls, movie theaters, Red Cross social and recreational canteens, officers' clubs, post exchanges, a post office, six operating rooms, a maternity ward, and glassed-in sun porches. The two post exchanges housed soda fountains, lunch counters, barber and beauty shops, libraries, tobacco counters, drug and sundry departments as well as retail merchandise. Two pharmacies, centrally located to all wards and clinics, filled as many as 60,000 prescriptions annually.

The hospital's physical therapy section was divided into four units, three of which were in Temple and one in Waco. They were outfitted with gymnasium equipment, devices to exercise amputation stumps, and a special foot apparatus for extremity elevation. Massage, hydrotherapy using whirlpool baths, resistance exercises, fever therapy, and electrical stimulation were techniques employed. McCloskey had its own shops for making artificial limbs, orthopedic braces, and other needed equipment and for fitting and training amputees with their prosthetic devices. Three experts in the brace shop fashioned the leather jackets and metal parts of artificial arms and legs. According to Colonel Bethea, "We could turn out a leg overnight if needed."[130] In 1945, the output of the brace shop numbered 3,920 braces, 1,611 limb prostheses, 2,817 shoe adjustments, and 1,394 canvas and leather belts and braces.[131] In August 1944, Captain Arthur M. Foust, the recruiting officer at McCloskey, announced the need for more personnel to work in the reconditioning program. According to Captain Foust, a plan had been worked out so that women might enlist in the Women's Army Corps and receive specialized training in educational reconditioning. Qualifications for this training required applicants to have a bachelor's degree as well as experience in teaching, newspaper or magazine writing, advertising, or social work. After basic training, enlistees received specialized training before being assigned to an army hospital.

McCloskey's Army Hospital Training Center, across the highway from the main installation, was the site where students and staff who were stationed in Temple lived and studied. A separate entity from the hospital, the temporary center had its own barracks, mess halls, and recreation halls. One of the first units to train was the 92nd General Hospital Unit with 500 men and 100 nurses.[132] They were stationed at McCloskey for an indefinite period. One notable trainee at McCloskey was Nora Staael, a student in the Mayo Clinic's new physical therapy

45

program. Staael joined the second class in July 1942, and the training program consisted of forty-four hours of class time per week for twenty-five weeks. Another six months of clinical training followed the classwork. Students were certified after one full year of training.[133] After completing their course work in December 1942, Staael and her classmates were sent to McCloskey General Hospital for six months of practical training. There they encountered polio patients, and Nora Staael adopted the controversial Sister Kenny method of treating the patients with hot packs and strenuous physical therapy. One incident revealed the resistance to this procedure:

> When she worked with her first polio patient at McCloskey General during the war, she knew exactly what to do. "Dr. James Scale told me," she later recalled, "to do what I did at Rochester. Then an orthopedic doctor came along and said, "That's malpractice!" because he was used to splinting [and immobilizing] patients."[134]

Nora Staael created quite a stir at McCloskey not only with her implementation of Kenny's work, but also with her outspoken dissatisfaction with the required uniforms. She found the pleated outfits with starched cuffs and collars unsuitable for handling patients. The physical therapists were also required to wear organdy "dusting caps" as Staael referred to them. She took it upon herself to redesign the uniform and dispense with the caps. In order to prevent administrators from reissuing the caps, Staael purchased the entire stock of organdy fabric in Temple and sent it home to her sisters in South Dakota.

When McCloskey opened in 1942, two dietitians were on duty: Edna E. Stinson from Walter Reed General Hospital and Beatrice Pearson, formerly of Scott and White Hospital.[135] Five more dietitians were expected. The larger cantonment hospitals generally had at least two enlisted patients' messes and an officer patients' mess. McCloskey had eight mess halls, and according to Captain John W. Cunningham, director of the hospital's dietetic division, approximately 13,450 meals were served daily. The food was prepared by 89 cooks, 45 of whom were civilians. Prior to mealtime, the hospital corridors were filled with men in maroon, moving along toward the mess hall directed by the mess sergeant. In the mess hall, some patients were served by waitresses while others filed through a self-service line, cafeteria style. There was no food rationing, but it was expected that no one would take more than he could eat. A sample menu for one day was as follows:

> **Breakfast:** oranges, dry cereal, whole wheat cereal, scrambled eggs or eggs to order,
> broiled bacon, jam, toast and butter, choice of beverage.
> **Dinner:** potato soup, barbecued chicken, honeyed sweet potatoes, whole kernel corn,
> green gage plum salad, mayonnaise, bread and butter, frosted brownies, choice of beverage.
> **Supper:** pork steaks, mashed potatoes, Dutch green beans, celery stuffed with pimento
> cheese, bread and butter, pineapple pie, choice of beverage.[136]

Everyone sat together at long tables covered with linen cloths. Officer patients sat apart from enlisted men in dining rooms where the linen-covered tables seated four. About one-third of the meals were served on the wards where kitchens were also located. Food brought from the main kitchen was re-heated and placed on individual serving trays.

Many hospitals had their own butcher shops and bakeries that served all mess halls. Gas ranges were most common, and some were equipped with grills. Gas or electric deep-fat fryers, mixers, vegetable steamers, kettles, mechanical vegetable peelers, coffee urns, rotary toasters, meat saws, slicers, grinders, and doughnut machines were standard issue in army hospitals. The hospital bakery produced 40,000 loaves of bread per month. With money from the Post Hospital Fund,

McCloskey purchased its own bread slicing and wrapping machine which was not only a sanitary and aesthetic improvement but a conservation measure as well. [137]

During the war, all named general hospitals had medical libraries. The War Department directed that libraries be supplied with current medical literature, and the Surgeon General's Office provided a selection of the most recently published books available. The amount and variety of books and periodicals furnished varied from library to library, depending on the medical specialties represented at the hospital, the size of the hospital, and its location. In addition to the books supplied by the Surgeon General's Office, each general hospital received a budget of $250 per year for the purchase of any additional books. The McCloskey Medical Library was in the main library and contained a wide variety of technical literature, medical journals, and medical textbooks available for use by the professional staff. [138]   In 1944, total holdings of the Medical Library were 634 books; 9,577 total volumes were held by all libraries.[139]

The completion of phase two of McCloskey added a branch library located on the upper floor of the second post exchange building. In addition to the new branch, there was a main library located over Post Exchange No. 1 and a branch in the Detachment Recreation Room. The new branch was equipped with furniture made at American Desk in Temple and with a collection of 2,000 books purchased for patient use. Rubber-tired carts, often in short supply, were used by the Red Cross to transport books to patients in the wards. Patient libraries were established with the goal of providing recreational reading to take the patient's mind off his illness and aid in his recovery. The therapeutic value of reading had been recognized by medical experts and was routinely employed as part of the patient's reconditioning and rehabilitation program. Educational materials assisted in developing new interests and optimism about returning to civilian life. Some libraries used a "book prescription" form on which the surgeon would suggest appropriate reading material for the patient as well as types to be avoided.

A laundry, steam plant, garage, and maintenance shops were essential to ensure proper functioning of all operations. The laundry alone employed 114 personnel who turned out 687,461 pieces of laundry per month including clothing of officers living in town.[140] Until the end of 1945, the post laundry also serviced the outside stations of Blackland Army Air Field, Waco Army Air Field, Temple Army Air Field, Hearne Internment Camp, and Mexia Internment Camp. By 1945, there were 150 employees working two shifts to process 1,463,169 individual pieces of laundry. A cleaning-pressing establishment was added to provide four-hour service for the hospital. The hospital's 'brig' or guard house was in the northeast corner away from all main buildings. Screened in steel wire, it had only two rooms and its own heating system.[141] A 500-seat chapel, offering interfaith services, was an important component, making McCloskey a self-contained community. It was the largest general hospital of the ten in the Eighth Service Command and one of the two largest in the country. Even as late as 1945, construction continued, and improvements were made to existing facilities. Most buildings were eventually air conditioned. One and one-half miles of sidewalks were laid, storm sewers were installed, a new library, W.A.C. barracks, and an addition to the brace shop were constructed, additional refrigeration was added to mess halls as well as a central meat-cutting room, roads were widened, and the water system was lengthened. Diving boards and ladders were added to the swimming pool, the most popular place at the hospital.

McCloskey was an integral part of the local community and maintained cordial relations throughout its existence. Electricity was bought from Texas Power and Light Company and gas from the Lone Star Gas Company in Temple. Water for all purposes was purchased from the City of Temple, and during 1945, an artesian well with the capacity to supply ordinary needs of the hospital was completed. Daily consumption of water from both the city and the well was estimated at 150 gallons per day per person.[142] The Hospital Dairy Farm in Temple supplied Grade-A pasteurized milk for the facility. Due to the shortage of milk in the area, additional milk was purchased from the Aerl Dairy in Waco and the Fort Worth Dairy Products Company in Fort Worth. The hospital had a contract with the Temple Dairy Products Company and Swift & Company of Temple for ice cream. The largest retail business in Temple was the hospital's Quartermaster Department store with an inventory of merchandise for 3,000 people. The store employed thirty-eight enlisted men and twenty-five civilian employees.[143]

The Chaplains Branch was active both on post and in the community. Colonel Bethea noted that the relationship between local clergy and the post chaplains was one of "splendid cooperation and helpfulness." Post chaplains often preached sermons in civilian churches and made presentations to civilian clubs and organizations. On post, they conducted religious services, visited patients in the wards and guardhouse, gave bedside devotions, distributed Bibles, handled welfare cases, and performed marriages, baptisms, and funerals.[144]

Tom Wright, former Temple fire chief, headed up the McCloskey fire department with 20 men on staff. Firemen were on duty 24 hours a day at the station where two fire engines were housed along with sleeping quarters for the men. The hospital also assisted Camp Hood in maintaining a Military Police presence of from eight to twenty men in the City of Temple as needed. They were provided from the guard section of the detachment.[145]

A contract post office was located on the reservation and managed by Miss Lola Winn, former postmistress at Parnell, Texas. Mail was sent twice daily from the Temple post office to McCloskey where it was sorted and taken to the proper wards, barracks, or offices six times per day. It functioned as other post offices and was authorized to sell war bonds and stamps, postage stamps, money orders, airmail envelopes, and package insurance. Telephone calls for McCloskey were routed through the telephone office in Temple where a team of operators worked to speed calls from patients to friends and relatives back home.

A civilian personnel office, under the supervision of Lieutenant Faraon J. Moss, handled all non-military, civil service employment at McCloskey. Moss was assisted by Miss Florence Anderson, chief clerk; Miss Catherine Tice, notary public; Miss Nona Shotwell, Miss Edna Black, Miss Anna L. Miller, Mrs. Bertha Johnson, and Marvin D. Coffman.[146] Civilians were hired when an enlisted man was not available for assignment. Age limits were raised for the duration of the war. In addition to employing personnel, the office kept injury reports, handled unemployment compensation, adjusted assignments as necessary, issued identification cards, provided counseling, and maintained personal files, leave records, and efficiency ratings for each employee.

Civilian women wore uniforms to make them readily identifiable. Since no national standard uniform for civilian women existed, McCloskey women could select their own. Approved by the commanding officer, the uniforms were pink khaki skirts with olive drab jackets, white blouses, and brown or black Oxfords with medium heels. An overseas-style cap matching the jacket completed the ensemble. Caduceus buttons worn on the uniforms were available at The Val-Art Shop and The Famous in Temple.

One of McCloskey's female civilian employees was quite unusual. In the early days, a stray mongrel dog appeared and became the hospital mascot and a permanent addition to the staff. Following is the story of Maggie McCloskey, written by Augustine Patison:

> A minor portion of McCloskey Army Hospital was ready for occupancy in 1942 and a small cadre of personnel moved in. A dozen or more dogs were then staying on the grounds; presumably, they had been abandoned by the former landowners. Within a month or so these dogs, with one exception, had wandered elsewhere in their

pursuit of happiness. One small pooch, now known as Maggie McCloskey, was quite content with the set-up and remained. To this day she has never left the reservation. She has no desire to roam the world and review its wonders; her universe begins and ends at McCloskey.

Maggie is part pointer, part just plain dog. Her hair is a sort of platinum blond with many dark spots. She is rather large, weighing a little more than a collie or shepherd. Formerly she was quite playful but nowadays she is full of dignity.
She liked adults but small children are a pain in the neck. She refuses to fraternize with them. In length of service she holds seniority over all employees of McCloskey Center; when this plant was opened officially late in 1942, Maggie was already an old timer.

Maggie has enjoyed the friendship of more soldiers and ex-soldiers than any other dog in the United States. She was a familiar sight to the multiplied thousands of service men whose destiny brought them to this hospital during the war years and the years subsequent thereto. For a long time, she fraternized daily with the many German prisoners of war who were in concentration at McCloskey, marching regularly with them to the mess hall. There is a large photograph of Maggie in the manager's office, and in all likelihood hundreds of snapshots of Maggie are in veterans' homes throughout the country.

At 6:00 a.m., Maggie meets the man who opens up No. 1 mess hall, goes in and eats breakfast, then takes a short post-breakfast nap. The meat man arrives to check in and Maggie accompanies him on his truck to get the day's supply of meat from the storage house. Finishing this task, she begins her job of patrolling the hospital's various corridors, wards, and offices. When feeling the urge to take a little snooze, she flops to the floor for a quick one, then resumes her work. At the noon hour she lines up with the wheelchair boys of No. 1 mess hall, escorts them to their dining room, and graciously remains to visit with them and accept a few choice handouts. After taking the first of her post-prandial siestas, Maggie resumes her patrol work, nearly always finishing in time to escort the wheelchair boys to supper. At night, she seeks diversion by attending ward parties or a recreation-hall picture show. (Patients swear to high heaven that she walks out on grade B pix if they are of the stinker category.) Her attendance at Sunday vesper services is highly commendable.

For a long time, Maggie was augmenting Temple's dog population with a new litter of puppies about every six months. It is in great part due to her that the local press has not found it necessary to alarm the citizenry with warnings of an impending canine shortage. One of our former doctors, possible deciding that Maggie deserved relief from the incessant trials and duties of motherhood, summoned a veterinarian for a professional service of some delicacy, and since then Maggie has heard no longer the pitter-patter of little feet. Her numerous progeny are widely dispersed through the Temple territory and all are leading exemplary lives. None has ever had a serious brush with the law.

It will be a grievous shock to many readers to learn that Maggie has a skeleton in her closet-- a gruesome, ghastly skeleton. Yes, this dignified old dowager once sowed some wild oats. When she was young and innocent, back in the days when military detachments were stationed at McCloskey, some of her soldier buddies began to tempt her with mugs of beer, available here at that time. For a while Maggie limited her libations to a short snort, just to be sociable.

But alas! Her short snorts became long snorts and soon she was guzzling double-headers with much joyful wagging of the caudal appendage. Her beer binges became frequent and her eyes became bleary. Her reputation suffered and her four-footed friends began to avoid her. She was definitely and irremissible in the doghouse. In the upper echelon of McCloskey canine circles, it was common gossip that Maggie had become a victim of the demon Suds and was perilously on the verge of becoming a barfly floozie.

Suddenly Maggie's life pattern changed radically. Possibly she had some colossal hangovers and stony-hearted nurses would give her nothing to relieve the jitters. Possibly her soldier pals chanced to note with much dismay that her bar bills were getting so high they were not the least big funny. Or possibly her inner strength of character manifested itself and she realized that not even a dog should go around mooching free drinks. Anyway, she became a staunch tee-totaler, and through these intervening years she had steadfastly remained a model of sobriety, exercising a fine and ennobling influence over all the other pooches of the community. Let us wistfully hope that this fine and ennobling influence extends also to all patients and domiciliary members of McCloskey VAC.

[Author's note: Maggie is dead now: died in convulsions after eating some poison-doped concoction that a mess hall employee had placed under one of the buildings for the purpose of destroying rodents. An employee directed the guards to bury Maggie down by the railroad tracks. Patients and domiciliary members protested so vociferously that her body was exhumed, placed in a neat little casket and buried in the center of a circular flower plot near the domiciliary barracks. One of the chaplains delivered a most eloquent oration relative to Maggie's loyalty and right living. Many a veteran in these United States still cherishes the memory of Maggie.][147]

The Waco annex had its own canine mascot named Wac, part bulldog and part mongrel. Wac accompanied patients on their walks but never went beyond the boundary of the property. On the first anniversary of the annex, Wac gave birth to eleven puppies which were so popular that all 320 patients wanted one![148]

Chapter 5: Home Away from Home

During World War II, the system for evacuation of the wounded from the front line to hospitals in the United States matured into an organized, structured system.[149] The army estimated that 80 to 90 percent of the wounded received first-aid treatment within an hour of being wounded. [150] After emergency care was provided in overseas field hospitals, patients were sent to evacuation hospitals where transportation arrangements were made. Generally, doctors were not consulted on the type of transportation patients received; however, in some cases, doctors were given a choice of plane or ship. Patients who required the attention of specialists were sent by plane; those requiring more general care were sent by boat. The choice was based entirely on a soldier's medical needs. A soldier's first stop would be a coastal debarkation hospital. After a stay of two to five days, patients were sent most often by train to a general or convalescent hospital with medical specialists to meet their unique needs and provide the necessary treatment. Every effort was made by the Medical Regulating Officer in Washington, D.C. to locate patients at hospitals closest to their homes. Most patients treated at McCloskey were transferred from other parts of the country or evacuated from overseas. Those coming to McCloskey from the Pacific Theater arrived via Letterman General Hospital in San Francisco; those from the European front were sent through Halloran General Hospital in New York.

The Medical Department had no trains on hand in 1939, but as the international situation deteriorated, the Corps of Engineers proposed a plan of implementing government-owned hospital trains. A study conducted by the army's Surgeon General showed that "unit cars" were more feasible, effective, and economical for use in the United States. The Office of the Surgeon General of the U.S. Army concentrated its efforts on developing plans for an ideal unit car. What followed were years of disagreements and compromises over the development of the ideal hospital train The army experimentation resulted in the following types of cars ultimately being implemented: ward cars containing berths to hold patients; ward dressing cars with clean areas to change dressings and perform emergency surgery; kitchen cars for food preparation and storage; and flexible unit cars with ward area, small kitchen and dressing room, a self-contained unit.[151] One hospital train normally had a capacity of 256 bed patients and was made up of sixteen ward cars, one utility car, one officer personnel car, two orderly cars, and one kitchen, dining, and pharmacy car. Electric and steam generators, storage lockers, food storage facilities, pharmacy, toilet facilities, sink, and medicine cabinets were on board. [152] By the end of the war, the army owned 202 unit cars, 80 ward cars, 38 ward dressing cars, and 60 kitchen cars for a total of 380 cars. [153]

During their travel to a general or convalescent hospital, returning soldiers received a War Department booklet that attempted to anticipate and answer questions about their medical care. *You're on Your Way.. HOME* explained how patients would be transported stateside and where. Each general hospital was listed with a description of its locale. A few details about Temple and McCloskey were briefly described:

> This hospital is located in Temple (pop. 15,344), Tex. (Lone Star State). Temple is widely known as a hospital center and seat of the Soil Conservation Program and is deep in the heart of Texas. In this region most of the population of the State is concentrated. Here also is found growing the State flower--the bluebonnet. Transportation from the city to the hospital is furnished by the Government-owned motor vehicles, commercial taxi service, and bus and rail service by Atchison, Topeka and Santa Fe Railway, and the Missouri-Kansas-Texas Railroad.[154]

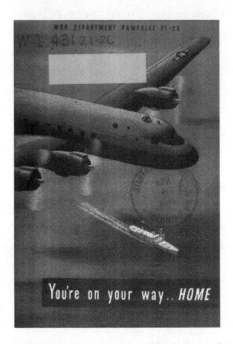

You're on your way.. HOME. War Department Pamphlet 21-26. Washington, D.C.: War Department, 1945. SOURCE: Internet Archive, public domain.

The booklet was helpful in providing details about laundry, visitors, entertainment, furloughs, chaplain services, discharge, and more for the soldier navigating his hospital stay. Furthermore, general expectations for physical reconditioning were enumerated. Another War Department pamphlet, *New Horizons*, explained the reconditioning program in more detail.[155] A series of classes was established so that patients could recover in progressive stages. Soldiers were told that an exercise program would begin even while they were confined to bed as Class IV patients; once they regained some strength and were classified as Class III patients, they would receive conditioning and remedial exercises using various sports such as volleyball, basketball, softball, and games. Class II patients showed more toughness with some slight weakness but were generally ready to resume the life of a soldier. Finally, Class I patients were those whose strength had returned and were able to spend eight hours a day toughening up to return to their outfits. The booklet went on to explain options in physical and occupational therapy and how these activities would speed the soldier's recovery.

Like other general hospitals, the focus at McCloskey was on healing the physical and psychological casualties of war. The hospital crest, seen on many hospital publications, featured a tree stump with branches and serpents and the phrase "Cui Proelia Sustinuit" meaning "For Him Who Has Fought the Battle." The tree stump represented the injured human body; the serpents represented the Medical Department. When the injured body came under the care of the Medical Department, new life, represented by green branches, sprang forth. Every branch of medicine was represented at the hospital including general medicine, general surgery, orthopedics, urology, plastic surgery, gastro-intestinal, neurosurgery, cardiology, dermatology, allergy, pathology, eye, ear, nose, and throat, psychiatry, X-ray, physical therapy, occupational therapy, dentistry, and other specialties. The hospital was equipped to handle all types of patients except for the blind, the deaf, and those requiring deep X-ray therapy. During 1944, McCloskey received designation as a Surgical Hospital which resulted in an enormous increase in surgical cases. A news story about medical care of patients at McCloskey provided a statistical breakdown of the types of cases being treated: in the medical division, 35% of the 1,200 patients were neuro-psychiatric cases, 12% were respiratory illnesses, 12% were gastro-intestinal problems, 7% arthritis, 6% heart disease; more than 50% of the 1,900 in the surgical division were orthopedic or amputation cases. Two-thirds of the patients were from overseas.[156]

In the early days, most McCloskey patients arrived at the hospital by train to the sound of a band playing. A spur from the Missouri-Kansas-Texas Railroad behind the hospital led to a covered enclosure where wounded soldiers were unloaded. Ambulatory patients were escorted to their assigned wards. Those on stretchers were off-loaded through train windows and taken by ambulance to their wards. In some instances, staff worked around the clock to unload and admit as many as five hundred patients per trainload. Upon arrival in Temple, the wounded were most often met by two medical officers: Lieutenant Colonel Sloan G. Stewart and Lieutenant Colonel Hannibal L. Jaworski, directors of the medical and surgical divisions, respectively. Jaworski remembered "many times that we would have twenty, thirty, or maybe even more planes land at Temple of these severely injured people so early after the initial procedures had been attempted or done, and that we could go on and proceed to take care of them." In July 1943, a group of 500 wounded from North Africa and the South Pacific arrived in Temple at one time followed by a group of German and Italian prisoners of war a month later. In October, two special trains brought in 700 patients at one time. In November, 125 wounded from Alaska and the Aleutian theaters of war reached McCloskey.

As time went on, air transport via C-47 army planes became the preferred method of evacuation, hitting a peak in July 1945 with 12,326 patients transported.[157] From January 1943 through November 1944, the number of patients arriving at Zone of Interior hospitals by air transport was about the same as the number arriving by sea. The planes were equipped with oxygen tents, blood plasma, and surgical equipment. General Kirk and other officers decided to test a plan for saving time in transporting seriously wounded patients from the seacoast to interior hospitals in anticipation of heavy demands once the invasion of Europe occurred. In January 1944, the army's first mass evacuation of wounded soldiers to a Zone of Interior hospital took place, and 75 wounded men were transported on three ambulance planes from a hospital ship at Charleston, South Carolina, to Temple.[158] The history-making, six-hour, 1,050-mile trip was successful and made travel faster and easier than railcars. Among the wounded were local men Jack G. White, Randall Wade, and August Waskow of Belton; A. L. Laughlin of Moody; and Jesse L. Stajanik of Little River. They were accompanied by army flight nurse, Lieutenant Madeline "Del" D'Eletto. Another large contingent of 375 ill and wounded from the South Pacific left San Francisco in May 1944 aboard twelve planes which distributed the soldiers among sixteen different hospitals with fifteen going to McCloskey.[159]   Their flight nurse, Lieutenant Jill Duskey, said the men sang "The Eyes of Texas" as the plane landed from stormy skies at the Temple Army Air Field. She said, "I'm from Wisconsin but I know all these Texas songs now."[160] Following the Normandy invasion in June 1944, the first four of many injured soldiers underwent a thirty-hour flight from Europe via Scotland to Temple, Texas. English hospitals were strained to the limit treating the wounded from the D-Day invasion.

McCloskey received many patients from the Pacific Theater with malaria. One newspaper article declared that "it takes about five minutes at the U.S. Army's largest hospital to discover that the principal concern of today's military medicine is malaria." [161] Colonel Bethea stated that his doctors were familiar with shrapnel, bullet, and bayonet wounds, but the bite of the anopheles mosquito was more problematic. Some patients were cured immediately while others had recurring cases. Colonel Stewart said, "We can stop the chills and fever, the worst of it, in 24 hours or so, but the disease keeps coming back. Tropical malaria is worse than we thought it would be." Lieutenant Colonel Paul Schmitt, chief of McCloskey's Laboratory Service, reported that malaria was the focus of research in Washington and other army medical centers, and although hopeful signs existed, none were the final solution. About 30 cases of filariasis, a tropical disease caused by a tiny parasitic worm, were also treated. The worm invaded the bloodstream and tissues, causing swelling of the glands. Colonel Stewart described the hospital as "the last court of appeal" for the patient, therefore making it imperative that medical staff devote conscientious study to each case. Each of the ten specialists available at McCloskey consulted on ten to fifteen cases daily. In some instances, as many as ten or twelve officers consulted on a single case. While it was not the norm, there were times when as many as 29 major operations were performed in a single day at McCloskey. This was possible only because McCloskey had a large recovery ward where patients were cared for by highly trained nurses. Air-conditioning in the summer months made patients' stays there even more comfortable.

As the returning men made their way to McCloskey, so did their families. A mini-invasion of sorts by friends and family armed with an abundance of home-cooked foods forced the hospital to issue a public appeal for sensible treatment of the sick. Hospital officials assured families that no effort was being spared to return their boys to health, but also warned that sick soldiers needed a period of treatment and convalescence which must play out scientifically and unemotionally. The bustle and flow of untold numbers of visitors interrupted the quiet atmosphere and goodies from home interfered with their regulated diets. Immediate family members could visit, but as the hospital stated, "A general hospital is no U.S.O."

Red Cross workers played an important part in serving as liaisons between patients and their families. When a patient was placed on the seriously ill list, the Red Cross sprang into action. A telegram was sent to the next of kin, and the Red Cross notified the patient's home chapter. The local Red Cross chapter discussed accommodations at McCloskey and relayed information about the family's mode of transportation and time of arrival in Temple. Families were met by a Red Cross social worker and escorted to the hospital. The social worker acted as hostess during the visit. The two Red Cross buildings at McCloskey accommodated 40 guests, free of charge. Meal tickets, costing 28 cents each, were available for purchase through the Post Exchange on weekdays and in the hospital mess hall on Sundays. Red Cross workers assisted with mail, long-distance phone calls, and any other needs. One of the officers' clubs made rooms available for wives of officer patients, limiting them to a fourteen-day stay in order to meet the need. Otherwise, families were encouraged to write detailed letters, full of fun, encouragement, and everyday activities to cheer up their loved ones. Plenty of letters were written with the McCloskey post office receiving an average of 80,000 letters, 3-4,000 newspapers, and 3,000 packages per month. Whether the hospital's gentle reprimand was heeded was unclear as in December 1943, *The Austin American-Statesman* reported "hundreds of parents, wives and other relatives of Camp Hood servicemen and the wounded at McCloskey General Hospital were flocking to town. Hotels were committed to full houses for the weekend. Trains and buses were packed, going and coming."

Unlike most other military hospitals, McCloskey had a full maternity ward with fourteen beds to serve expectant soldiers' wives. A news story in July 1943 reported that the maternity ward was at full capacity with fifteen infants.[162] Red Cross volunteers from Bell County were on hand to supply new mothers with baby gifts and other necessities. The first baby born at McCloskey was Stephen Hetzler, son of Lieutenant and Mrs. Stanley A. Hetzler. [163] He was born November 2, 1942, delivered by Hannibal "Doctor Joe" Jaworski, a surgeon from Waco who had been assigned to McCloskey.[164] Following the birth, General Bethea notified the army's Surgeon General that McCloskey had its first delivery. One year later, the hospital honored Hetzler with a birthday party. The invited children played games and were served individual small cakes and ice cream. In 1945, 185 male babies and 204 female babies were born at the hospital; there were four sets of twins.[165]

One of the harsh realities of World War II was the high rate of mental casualties. Factors contributing to this were the mental strain related to extensive periods of offensive action, the increased fury of modern warfare, and low morale. After the war, two leading psychiatrists argued that one of the most important lessons of World War II was that it required psychiatrists "to shift attention from problems of the abnormal mind in normal times to problems of the normal mind in abnormal times." [166] The number of neuropsychiatric disorders was reported to be "two to three times that of World War I despite the fact that rejections for psychiatric reasons were five to six times greater than those of World War I."[167] The army was unprepared to deal with the large number of neuro-psychiatric cases. A shortage of professional personnel exacerbated the problems.

On August 5, 1944, McCloskey was officially designated as a Psychiatric Center for closed-ward patients, and shortly thereafter as a Neurological Center.[168] The neuropsychiatric division was headed up by Lieutenant Colonel Guy C. Randall who had been associated with the Massachusetts State Hospital prior to the war. In 1943, Randall reported that two-thirds of the 6,410 medical diagnoses made at the hospital were sent there because of nervous disorders. During the first part of the war, most patients arriving from overseas were open-ward patients; that changed in 1944 when the preponderance of admissions were psychotic patients. The most serious patients were housed in closed wards at the south end of the section for mental cases.[169] The men in the closed wards were those who developed mental disorders from startling circumstances or a chain of events in battle. Electroencephalography was a useful tool for recording brain activity and helping the physician obtain a complete history of the patient. Treatments offered at McCloskey included sodium amytal narcosynthesis, electric shock therapy, pneumoencephalography, myelograms, spinal taps with dynamics, and hydrotherapy, using the continuous bath and wet sheet packs to relax mentally disturbed patients. Hypnotism was used to help patients regain their memories. One such soldier lost his memory after a certain point in the Battle of Salerno. Another boy "froze" with machine guns firing overhead.

Colonel Sloan Stewart suggested that only a small percentage of the cases were true mental illness. According to Stewart, most were persons with exaggerated nervous conditions which could be treated with occupational and recreational therapy. Most patients had their entire day planned with exercise, group therapy, and "industrial" or occupational therapy as part of the routine. Early on, the army found that soldiers responded more positively to their treatments if they kept their minds and hands busy by accomplishing something rather than simply lying in bed. Occupational therapists used craft projects and model building to reduce hospital fatigue, to foster confidence, and to offer another form of exercise. Fifteen percent of the neuropsychiatric patients discharged from McCloskey were able to return to active duty.

The number of patients continued to increase even as the war slowed in 1945. To handle the patient load from overseas, emergency beds were set up in the main hospital. Almost 300 veterans from nearly every battlefront poured into McCloskey in June 1945 on three large train convoys. To greet them, the McCloskey Band played "Deep in the Heart of Texas" while the maimed and wounded clapped as they were able. All the arrivals were in high spirits despite wounds and injuries. Among them were 2nd Lieutenant Wilma Dobias of St. Johns, Michigan who had served 14 months in New Guinea. From Clarita, Oklahoma, came Private First Class Samuel D. Nelson who had been shot in the leg by a Hitler youth. Texas was represented by Marvin Tunnicliff of Denton who had lost an eye and received a fractured skull at the Maginot Line.

In July 1945, it was reported that McCloskey had admitted 34,033 bed patients in two years. At McCloskey beds were spaced only a foot apart, and the hospital was nearly at full capacity most of the time. The number of average patient days was 60 in 1944 and 81 in 1945.[170] General Bethea said, "We had a total of 4,600 beds, and at one time had 5,600 patients on the rolls. No, we didn't have two in a bed, but rather had about fifteen hundred or more on furlough or sick leave."[171] Throughout the war, many patients received medals and other forms of decoration and recognition during their hospital stays. McCloskey also treated soldiers from Camp Hood and from Camp Swift in Bastrop, the largest army training and transshipment camp in Texas. During World War II, Camp Swift housed a maximum strength of 90,000 troops and 3,865 German prisoners of war.[172] The mortality rate at McCloskey was "remarkably low" considering the large numbers of patients being cared for.[173] Forty-four deaths were recorded for 1944 and 47 for 1945.[174] Between 25 and 50 patients received certificates of disability discharges daily and returned to civilian life. Others returned to active duty.

With the capitulation of Japan in August 1945, it was expected that there would be a large turnover of civilian employees at McCloskey. Captain John C. Hamilton, director of the Personnel Division, reported no change in the number of resignations among civilians. For the previous two months, McCloskey was at its peak with casualties arriving daily.

Chapter 6: Beyond Affliction

On June 1, 1943, Major General Norman T. Kirk succeeded Major General Magee as Surgeon General of the U.S. Army, appointed by President Franklin D. Roosevelt. [175] Prior to becoming the Surgeon General, Major General Kirk, a renowned orthopedic surgeon, was assigned first to Walter Reed Hospital and then to General Hospital No. 3 in Colonia, New Jersey, to care for the large number of World War I casualties arriving home from France in 1918-1919. It was a complex process that included planning the treatment and evacuation of soldiers through successive military facilities as well as their wound care en route to a more stabilized environment like the amputation center. During his time at the two amputation centers, Major General Kirk studied 1,700 patients with amputations and operated on more than 700 of them, subsequently publishing a monograph entitled *Amputations, Operative Techniques* in 1924. [176] One insight he gained was that most surgeons were unaware of factors that affected patients' outcomes. His experiences allowed him to observe amputees through the process of wound closure, stump healing, and initial prosthetic fitting.[177] Care of the amputee was, in Kirk's opinion, a straightforward process: produce a good residual limb for better prosthetic fitting which in turn would provide improved function and ambulation for the patient. [178] To achieve this outcome, he recommended "open circular" amputation in which the surgeon performed the surgery at the lowest level of viable tissue and closure of the residual limb once it met certain clinical and bacterial biopsy criteria. For closure, he advised three procedures: a simple plastic closure, a myodesis with plastic closure, and revision amputation to the next higher level. He did not recommend the use of skin grafts to close the residual limb because of the lack of sensation in the graft. Sensation was important since the skin bore weight through the prosthesis. By 1938, Kirk foresaw the looming threat of war and realized that patients with limb loss would require specialized care. He became the first U.S. Army physician to become board certified in orthopedic surgery.[179]

Once he became U.S. Army Surgeon General, Kirk implemented his amputation care protocols to provide consistent medical care. Rather than leaving decision-making to individual practitioners, it was his goal to establish fast, efficient, and consistent care for patients across the board who had a variety of doctors during the stages of amputation, wound care, and prosthetic fitting. As soon as new improvements were recognized, he put them into action. In 1944 prior to the arrival of large numbers of wounded from Europe, Kirk requested a review of all amputee centers by civilian consultants to identify problem areas. A second review was done in October 1945, and both reports praised the high quality of care given to amputees despite personnel and equipment shortages.[180] Two problems identified were the waiting times for prostheses as well as the types of prostheses needed for young, active patients. During World War II, prostheses were a definite problem and studies were conducted to improve both temporary and permanent prostheses. Researchers experimented with different materials including plastic, Bakelite, and various metals, and conducted investigations on gait and prosthetic/residual limb interface.[181] Of the soldiers in the U.S. Army wounded during World War II, about 15,000 required major amputations, and more than 90% were cared for at amputee centers after the invasion of Europe in June 1944.[182] Of the amputees who arrived in the Zone of Interior hospitals, about 20% were upper extremity and 80% lower extremity losses.[183] In World War I, amputations above the knee were most numerous, but the situation reversed in World War II. In World War II, one amputee in every twenty lost two extremities and less than one in every 200 experienced a hip joint amputation.[184] Credit was given to improved surgical competence. Statistics obtained from reports from amputation centers showed a breakdown in types of amputation with single amputations at 13,844 (one leg, 10,620 or 1 arm, 3,224), double amputations at 927 (both legs, 870 or both arms, 57), and triple amputations at 9 (both legs and one arm, 8, or both arms and one leg, 1).[185]

The chart below showed the end-of-quarter census of amputees at U.S. Army amputation centers from 30 June 1944 to 31 March 1946 including McCloskey General Hospital:

TABLE 14.—*Number of admissions*[1] *to U.S. Army amputation centers, January 1943–December 1945*

[Preliminary data based on reports from amputation centers]

Center	January 1943–April 1944		May 1944–December 1945		January 1943–December 1945	
	Number of amputees	Number of stumps	Number of amputees	Number of stumps	Number of amputees	Number of stumps
Bushnell General Hospital	203	217	2,043	2,160	2,246	2,377
England General Hospital		[2]	2,106	2,251	2,106	2,251
Lawson General Hospital	241	252	1,942	2,075	2,183	2,327
McCloskey General Hospital	271	284	2,339	2,476	2,610	2,760
McGuire General Hospital		[3]	735	780	735	780
Percy Jones General Hospital	367	382	2,494	2,681	2,861	3,063
Walter Reed General Hospital	588	624	1,825	1,963	2,413	2,587
Total	1,632	1,718	12,926	13,782	14,558	15,500

[1] Admissions for major amputations. Data for each center include cases transferred from another amputation center; total includes new cases only.
[2] England General Hospital was established in August 1944.
[3] McGuire General Hospital was established in March 1945.

Source: Medical Statistics Division, Surgeon General's Office, Department of the Army, 14 Oct. 1955.

The War Department aided amputees by distributing a booklet entitled *"Helpful Hints to Those Who Have Lost Limbs."* It included information on the care of the stump, phantom pain, adapting to prostheses, and other questions common to amputee patients. The booklet introduced patients to Charles McGonegal who lost both arms in World War I, showing him engaged in everyday activities using mechanical hooks for hands. McGonegal was also featured in an educational film entitled *Meet McGonegal*, encouraging soldiers to live independently even with a prosthesis.[186] McGonegal demonstrated shaving, hair combing, tying shoelaces, dressing, eating breakfast typing, talking on the telephone, and even smoking a cigarette! At a showing of the film in Austin, A. O. Williams, Texas service officer, expressed his desire that relatives, businessmen, and prospective employers of amputees would turn out to view the film to aid their understanding and

69

acceptance of soldiers who had lost a limb. As Williams said, "After all the amputee's greatest handicap is -- you and I. The rest of us need readjustment as bad or worse than he does." [187]

The Surgeon General promoted the idea of training of amputees by amputees, and many amputees traveled around the country visiting patients in hospitals showing them how they had learned to adapt to army-built legs or arms. Charles McGonegal was paid a stipend for his services to the military and veterans' hospitals. He visited McCloskey in July 1945 and the mere sight of him "handling the complicated-looked array of hooks and clamps that serve for hands is worth a million assurances that everything is going to be all right." The Honorable Richard Wood, the son of Lord Halifax, the British ambassador to the United States, was a double leg amputee from injuries sustained when a German dive bomber planted a bomb in his lap in North Africa. Although the bomb was a dud, it crushed his legs which had to be amputated above the knees. He made a nation-wide tour of military hospitals in the United States to visit with other amputees. "The boys in the hospitals need to see veterans who have undergone their handicap," he pointed out. "Although people told me I would be able to walk perfectly well with artificial legs, it would have picked me up for someone to walk in and show me," he said.[188] The Englishman, who entertained the Texas House and Senate chambers, spoke seriously of the rehabilitation problems of returning service men. "After touring American military hospitals, I have found that rehabilitation efforts for wounded veterans have been excellent. When I went through McCloskey Hospital, I was especially pleased. As a matter of fact, the boys there actually cheered me up." Many lifelong friendships developed among the men who often spent months recuperating in the hospital and learning to use their prosthetics. In 1949, Don Beaton, a former McCloskey patient, made good on his promise of "I'll be seeing you" to his wartime buddies from the "Amputee Club" on Ward 119-A. From their home in Fargo, North Dakota, Don and his wife made a 3,500-miles trip to visit nine other men who made their homes in various parts of the country after being discharged from McCloskey. Among those he planned to see were Bruce Matison, who worked as a rural mail carrier in Mankato Minnesota, and Tom Steensland of Austin, Texas, who was employed in radio advertising and had married a McCloskey nurse.[189]

Early in the war, amputation stumps were placed in traction until healed and ready for surgery. Later it was determined that physical therapy aided in the healing of the stump, and the type of therapy most often used to relieve pain, increase circulation, and form granulation tissue was a whirlpool bath. Some amputation centers employed the use of stump massage. Once surgery was done, the amputee began a physical therapy regimen designed for each patient's individual needs to "strengthen weak muscles, stretch contractures, and to shape the stump."[190] Proper bandaging of the stump was crucial and physical therapists taught amputees how to manage their own bandages with mixed results. Major General Kirk told a news reporter that all artificial limbs were purchased by the government from a firm in Minneapolis, Minnesota for an average cost of $42 each.[191] Most often the delay was in getting the stump ready to receive the limb.

The next step was learning to use prostheses. Patients with an amputation of the lower extremity were taught to walk by the physical therapist while patients with an upper extremity amputation were trained in the use of a mechanical hook by the occupational therapist. For walking instruction, amputees were classified according to their disability into four groups: unilateral above knee, unilateral below knee, hip disarticulation, and bilateral. [192] The patients, most of whom were young, healthy soldiers, were highly motivated to get back on their feet and become productive civilians. Upon receipt of their prostheses, the men, dressed in swim trunks, would start on crutches as the physical therapist checked their balance, speed, and fit, always looking for blisters or areas of discomfort. Once patients advanced to the intermediate class, crutches were exchanged for canes and emphasis was placed on developing rhythm and stride. It was essential that the physical therapist correctly assess problem areas and correct them so the patient could walk properly.

At the end of the course, patients were required to pass an achievement test that included such activities as falling and getting up, stepping on and off a curb, climbing a hill, and walking on rough terrain. Men with artificial hands had to master many practical life skills such as playing checkers, throwing a ball, driving a nail, using a saw, lacing their shoes, buttoning their shirts, folding a letter, shaving, opening a door, using brooms and garden tools, and lighting a match. Their graduation came with eating in the mess hall and successfully demonstrating use of a cup, spoon, knife, and fork. One of the best stories about the perseverance of amputees came from McCloskey:

> [The patient] was fitted out with an artificial limb and had learned to use it well enough that he made a Saturday night date with some fair damsel of the town. But his new leg developed a mechanical hitch and had to be sent back to the factory. Nothing daunted, our hero borrowed a leg from another patient. It was several inches shorter than his, however. After limping around the room a few times, the kid burst out: "Why, I can't go out like this--somebody might think I was a cripple!" [193]

Competitive games and sports were important for both physical and psychological rehabilitation. Players often became so interested in the game they temporarily forgot about their physical limitations. McCloskey had its own volleyball, baseball, softball, and basketball teams, and regularly engaged teams from other hospitals and military installations in the Eighth Service Command. The McCloskey basketball team gained notoriety for its skilled moves in scoring, blocking, and ball handling that frustrated the opposition. Forming an 18-man team called the Purple Hearters, the boys rotated six-man playing groups with three forwards and three guards. Because the team was made up of patients with newly acquired artificial limbs, they played by girls' rules and were willing to take on any five-member female team. Most of the boys had never played against women before and soon discovered the women were no pushovers. Their undefeated status led team captain, Allen S. Monts, of Charleston, Illinois, to issue a challenge to play any girls team in the nation. Locally, the Purple Hearters defeated the WACS, nurses, and cadet nurses who were the champs of the Temple Women's Basketball League. Feeling their oats, Monts said, "We could give any of them a good game although we have to work harder now than when we had our limbs and played good five-man teams." Their coach was Captain Clyde T. Jetton of Salina, Oklahoma, whose right leg was amputated above the knee. The top scorers were Private First Class Jack L. Ryder (Nebraska City, NE.) and Private First Class Clarence Montgomery (Los Angeles, CA.) Other players on the team were Charles S. Ramsey (Mansfield, LA.); Pete A. Ochoa (Galveston, TX.); Erwin L. Moore (Caldwell, TX.); Edward L. Pace (Monticello, AR.); Bill Weidler (Ocheyedan, IA.); Harold Kneller (Fort Wayne, IN.); and Arvie Walker (Lufkin, TX.).

The McCloskey softball team was quite skilled, often advancing to district and championship finals. In August 1944, McCloskey and Fort Bliss entered the softball finals. The Eighth Service Command's softball championship tournament was held in Dallas with Camp Gruber battling Jackson Barracks in the initial contest, and McCloskey battling Red River Ordnance Plant in the second. The winner played Fort Sam Houston and Fort Bliss. McCloskey advanced to the semi-finals, taking on Fort Bliss, and then to the finals against Fort Sam Houston for the five-state honor. The tourney was won by Fort Sam Houston which downed McCloskey 4-2.[194] Again in 1945, McCloskey defeated the Eighth Service Command Headquarters team to move into the semi-finals against Camp Wolters. The finals were scheduled to be held in Temple August 8-11, 1945 but were cancelled by the Eighth Service Command due to transportation issues.

McCloskey's wheelchair baseball garnered national attention in an article in *The New York Times* that credited the wounded soldiers at the hospital with inventing the game.[195] "Baseball on wheels has been developed here by war veterans who refuse to give up their favorite sport just because they have lost arms or legs." A tennis court served as a diamond with eight players using a regulation bat and volleyball. Members of the wheelchair baseball league included Stanley Heck (Chicago, IL.); W. R. Hanna (Sioux City, IA.); Leo Michelson (Chicago, IL.); Clarence Powell (Fort Worth, TX.); Bill Moomey (Muscatine, IA.); Willard L. Fox (Tulsa, OK.; James Driscoll (Dubuque, IA.); Warren Bradbury (Tulsa, OK.); and Robert Collett (Pineville, KY.).[196]

Poor planning in the construction of many general hospitals often resulted in therapy clinics that were too small to handle the heavy workload of thousands of patients with major amputations. Such was not the case at McCloskey. Occupational therapy was concentrated in a building of its own with specialty rooms including a gymnasium, leather shop, carpenter shop, pottery room, two printing rooms, an art room, and weaving

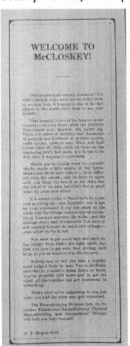

room. The craft shops were not designed to teach the men a trade but to provide them with worthwhile activities to pass the time while they healed. Its robust program of occupational therapy expanded each year. In 1945, four new shops were added with ten graduate therapists, eight apprentices, nine civilians, and four enlisted men staffing the department. A comprehensive therapeutic program for paraplegic patients was inaugurated.[197]

Occupational therapy included activities such as making camouflage netting (to recover the use of stiff shoulder muscles), molding clay (to loosen injured joints or tendons), operating a foot-powered saw (to recover flexibility in a stiff knee), or playing chess or checkers (to adapt to an artificial arm or hand). One activity that was especially popular with bed patients was clay modeling. It provided corrective therapy by strengthening arm, wrist, and leg muscles in throwing the clay, turning the hand wheel, and working the kick and treadle wheels. Miss Carolyn Phillips, a graduate of Mary Hardin-Baylor College and therapist aid, served as the instructor in charge of clay modeling and assisted patients in creating pottery items such as sets of dishes, mugs, souvenir plates, busts, costume jewelry, and belt buckles. All the large ashtrays in the hospital corridors were created by the pottery students. [In 2020, a pottery vase made at McCloskey was listed for auction on Ebay].

In 1944, Miss Edna Vehlow, senior therapist at McCloskey, presented a program for the Lions' Club to show off handmade articles of leather, felt, and wood created by patients in the occupational therapy program. Captain Richard Green, Chief of Occupational Therapy, reported that leather work was the most popular activity followed by weaving. In December 1945, McCloskey's Building 51 had the appearance of Santa's workshop as the patients turned out handmade leather billfolds and purses, hobby horses, table lamps, brightly colored rugs, ashtrays, toys, and many other items for Christmas gifts. Bookends, bowls, and vases were created at the pottery shop. Miss Vehlow reported that 1,800 convalescent patients participated in the program, and within two weeks, 642 ambulatory patients had made 3,210 articles. [198] The value of leather goods alone was estimated at $22,420 retail. In the photographic laboratory, Private First Class Leroy J. Miller of Highwood, Illinois, assisted patients with portraits for their families. Captain Green summed up by saying, "It's mighty good medicine."

Hospital work such as dusting, cleaning floors, pushing food carts, and washing windows, was often assigned to encourage physical activity. McCloskey allowed patients (and later domiciliary members) could have their own gardens where they grew easy-to-harvest vegetables such as corn, peas, tomatoes, and okra. The *Texas Farm News* reported a mile-long row of green beans running the full-length of the fence surrounding the hospital.[199] Ambulatory patients were selected to be hospital guides, providing tours for visitors and relating first-hand information on the details of hospital life. Most of the twenty hospital guides had lost arms or legs but were sufficiently ambulatory to perform the task. Corporal Herman Hein of Bellaire, Ohio, said, "It's the most interesting and best job I've done since I've been a patient here." Others selected for guide duty were James E. Adams (Springfield, IL.), Louis R. Cabrera (Los Angeles, CA.), William B. Dobbins (Kilgore, TX.), Alfred E. Dolynko (Detroit, MI.), Neal S. Ford (El Paso, TX.), Clayton A. Ford (Laconia, NH.), Archie B. Freeman (Clinton, OK.), Woodrow W. Hardy (Oklahoma City, OK.), Gordon Oliphant (Waco, TX.), Elmer L. Oliver (New Haven, IL.), Emmett V. Smith (San Antonio, TX.), Luther E. Spears (New Braunfels, TX.), Tom F. Starr (Ballinger, TX.), Maynard C. Theobald (Peoria, IL.), Clifton C. Whitley (Corsicana, TX.), William C. Clifford (Camden, NJ.), Herbert L. Dawson (Tuckerman, AR.), Tommy Boswell (Hughes, AR.), and John B. Schwager (Blue Earth, MN.)[200]

Music was another aspect of the reconditioning program at McCloskey, having been made an official part of the army's program in October 1943. Surgeon General Kirk and other military officials recognized the effect music had on troop morale and its importance for the wounded men. While it was not initially referred to as "music therapy," it served the same therapeutic purpose by being incorporated into the Red Cross recreation programs. As time went on, the War Department contemplated implementing musical therapy programs in hospitals. In April 1944, Lieutenant Lester L. Rankin, music and entertainment officer at McCloskey and Sergeant Nathan H. Shanks attended the Texas Federation of Music Clubs Convention in Houston. They attended sessions to observe how musical therapy might be applied to the hospital.

In 1945, the War Department's Technical Bulletin *Music in Reconditioning in ASF Convalescent and General Hospitals* was published "to set forth a program of music in reconditioning and to present methods and techniques of presentation of music to patients convalescing in Army hospitals." Furthermore, the benefits of music were enumerated,

> Music should be provided along with other activities offered to patients because it is one of the most effective vehicles for bringing & group together, for releasing the emotions, and for creating a spirit of fellowship and esprit de corps. If the patient is an individual performer, music provides an opportunity for self-expression, accomplishment, and. satisfaction. If he is a group performer, he will establish contacts with others mutually interested. If he simply listens to music, his interests are broadened, and his sense of wellbeing is generally increased. In neuropsychiatric treatment sections, a well-rounded program of musical activities is especially desirable. The response of neuropsychiatric patients on closed wards to music activities may be slow at first. However, under skillful guidance, it is possible to increase this response until most patients are deriving social. and mental benefits through their interest in music.[201]

A music department was inaugurated at McCloskey in September 1944.[202] Professional music teachers were selected, the music room organized, four practice rooms set up, and lessons scheduled. During the last three months of the year, 276 lessons were given. A musical instrument library with 74 instruments available for loan to patients was heavily used.

Patients at McCloskey participated in dances, musical parties, talent shows, and sing-a-longs, and enjoyed musical programs by various school groups and entertainers. On Saturday nights, dances were held in the gymnasium with

Temple girls and Mary Hardin-Baylor College coeds in attendance.

In 1943, McCloskey was granted use of the National Youth Administration Center in Waco for reconditioning and training of amputees with skills necessary for civilian life. The "Waco Annex," as it was called, was located on thirty-two acres northwest of the Circle and commanded by Captain Packard Thurber. It had a dormitory capacity of 320 beds, a mess hall for 260, a gymnasium, and post exchange. In instances where men were waiting for weeks to see if a bone graft or other procedure was successful, they were sent to Waco to learn a trade. The average stay was four to six weeks. The shops on site were equipped for teaching patients to be electricians or carpenters or automotive repair technicians. An ordnance shop offered patients an opportunity to train and qualify to advance to the army's ordnance shop in Austin as an apprentice upon discharge from the hospital. Men were taught to drive, take public transportation, go horseback riding and swimming. General Bruce's daughter, Linnell, devoted much of her time to working with patients there.[203] The Department of Public Safety partnered with McCloskey in providing the opportunity for soon-to-be-discharged amputees to take driver's license examinations and driving tests. A few modifications were made to assist the men in driving such as steering knobs or stirrups and springs on the clutch or accelerator. Ability to pass the test restored the patients' confidence before they resumed life in the real world.

Major General Kirk wanted to see for himself that quality care was being provided for soldiers, so he regularly toured and inspected amputation centers. In August 1943, he arrived in Temple to review operations at McCloskey General Hospital.[204] Unbeknownst to Kirk, McCloskey surgeon, Colonel Hannibal "Doctor Joe" Jaworski had pioneered the ideas of early ambulation following surgery and the use of elastic stockings and described how it happened:

I started early ambulation in McCloskey General Hospital with the okay and the blessings of General Bethea. We had received many hernia operations and many other operations. We got them up, if possible, the very next day. The rule and the instructions were that they must stay in bed a week, then go home for a week or two and recuperate... I really don't have any evidence of early ambulation being instituted in any of the larger hospitals...This was, I believe, sort of a project of my own, a belief of my own, which was encouraged later by several of my good friends, by my associates, and especially General Bethea. He and I believed very strongly in early ambulation, and it was very fine for me to have a man of his caliber to stand behind my early thoughts and my early beliefs. [205]

Jaworski claimed that early ambulation made his patients the "happiest ones on the hall." Even the maternity patients were involved in the practice of early ambulation. In his career Jaworski had observed many patients who died suddenly from pulmonary embolism as a result of being confined to bed. Jaworski would not take credit for the innovation of elastic stockings: "Well, it was not really all my innovation, it was probably brought about by several of us who looked for anything to improve the circulation because we knew it was circulatory change that brought about these bad aftereffects." [206] Before elastic stockings became widely available, elastic bandages were used. It was routine for post-operative and post-delivery patients to wear elastic stockings for several days. When the Surgeon General arrived and began to question the patients on the surgical wards, Jaworski recounted Kirk's reaction in his memoirs:

He immediately turned to me and said he wanted to talk to me. He said, "What are you doing? You should have read the orders that they should stay in bed for at least a week." About that time, General Bethea spoke up and said, "Colonel Jaworski has started an early ambulation here at our hospital with my consent. You would be surprised at the happiness that these boys have shown by being able to get up and move about."[207]

Kirk later told General Bethea, the commander of McCloskey, "We have to get this young surgeon out of here. His ideas have not proven at all." General Bethea persuasively argued in favor of Jaworski's methods, and Kirk eventually approved the use of early ambulation on all patients. Colonel Jaworski summed up the results of Kirk's visit:

> I think, knowing Surgeon General Kirk, being a man of vast experience and also a man who believed in new ideas, that he began to study this problem, and when he saw the good results, he was proud to start this program then in the large hospitals. This was part of my greatest success while in the army. [208]

Initially, Jaworski was hesitant to share his methods with other physicians until the benefits were proven. Jaworski shared his ideas with other medical professionals, and they were well-received by doctors from around the area. Jaworski believe early ambulation saved lives:

> I could truthfully say, and I believe that I am right, that seventy-five percent of post-operative and post-delivery cases, seventy-five percent of the aftereffects and the changes that resulted from staying in bed too long, were completely abolished. [209]

In January 1945, McCloskey was selected as one of two general hospitals in the Eighth Service Command to host a three-day conference featuring Dr. Sterling Bunnell, a civilian orthopedic consultant to General Kirk.[210] Dr. Bunnell established the specialty of hand surgery during World War II. The intensive schedule included instructing and demonstrating surgical procedures on the hand, round-table discussions, and review and examination of patients.

The Surgeon General visited Temple again in October 1945 on a two-day inspection tour. He was accompanied by Rep. Iver D. Fenton, member of the House Military Affairs Committee, and Brigadier General W. Lee Hart, surgeon of the Eighth Service Command. The Temple Chamber of Commerce honored the distinguished guests with a dinner at the Kyle Hotel. The *Belton Journal* reported that "progress in perfecting artificial arms and legs for amputees is one of [Kirk's] special interests.[211] The Consultant in Orthopedic Surgery from the Surgeon General's Office also made inspection tours. In one program evaluation, the following observation was made,

> At some hospitals, such as Ashburn (McKinney, Tex.) and McCloskey (Temple, Tex.) General Hospitals, medical officers and physical therapy technicians showed a gratifying knowledge of their patients' needs and status. At a few other hospitals, where personnel was equally adequate and equipment was in equally good supply, the reverse was true. It was not strange that the results in the first mentioned hospitals were excellent while those in the second group ranged from fair to poor.[212]

Civilian consultants to the Surgeon General made a second inspection of amputation centers in October 1945. The physicians made their visits as members of the Committee on Prosthetic Devices in addition to their roles as consultants. Their report confirmed previous opinions of the high quality of the surgical treatment and prosthetic fitting amputees received. "It should be pointed out that the Army had to prepare organized services for an unknown number of amputees. We feel that exceptional commendation is due [to] the Surgeon General and the Medical Department of the Army for having successfully handled an emergency problem the like of which had never previously been encountered in modern times."[213] It was announced in 1946 that McCloskey General Hospital was designated as a research center for the improvement of artificial limb joints in below-knee amputations. The Surgeon General's Office allocated $44,000 for experimental research and provided ten enlisted men to staff a newly equipped building.[214]

The people of Temple were reminded daily of the high cost of war as hospital patients could circulate freely in the community. On one day Walter Humphrey, editor of the *Temple Daily Telegram*, observed as many as 37 amputees within four blocks as he walked from his newspaper office to the post office. Humphrey found it reassuring that the people of Temple did not stare at the armless and legless men but rather offered friendly greetings as they passed on the streets. He wrote a story which was carried nationwide about the high morale of the amputees at McCloskey:

> The people of Temple join the doctors and attendants at McCloskey Hospital in making one claim you can't talk them out of. That is, that the amputee has better morale than any other man in or out of the Army. The morale in the hospital's amputation wards is phenomenal. It is genuinely contagious. In no other part of the big 4,000-bed hospital is the morale as good. These amputees are the hospital's biggest kidders, its most inveterate pranksters, its liveliest patients. You can't make a tour of McCloskey's corridors without running onto a couple of crippled men trying to outrun each other on their crutches... or

a man cutting traffic capers in his wheelchair. A lost leg or a lost arm... or both. It isn't getting the American soldier down. He's still got his fighting heart and his sense of humor, and the best artificial limbs science can provide. He's getting set for a job in civilian life and nothing can stop him. His morale is 100 percent. He doesn't want sympathy. He just wants a chance to make good when he sheds his uniform and dons civvies again. And from the way he talks, nothing can stop him.[215]

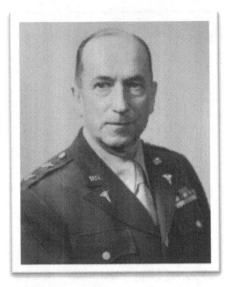

James Albertus Bethea, Commanding Officer of McCloskey General Hospital, 1942-1946.
SOURCE: Wikimedia Commons, public domain.

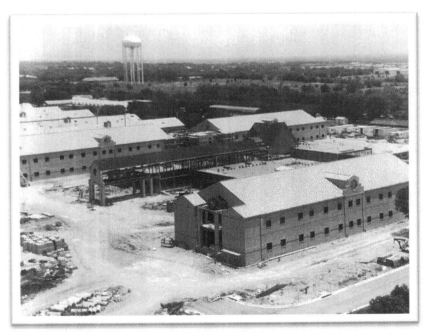

McCloskey General Hospital under construction, 1942.
SOURCE: Olin E. Teague Veterans' Center Medical Library Archives.

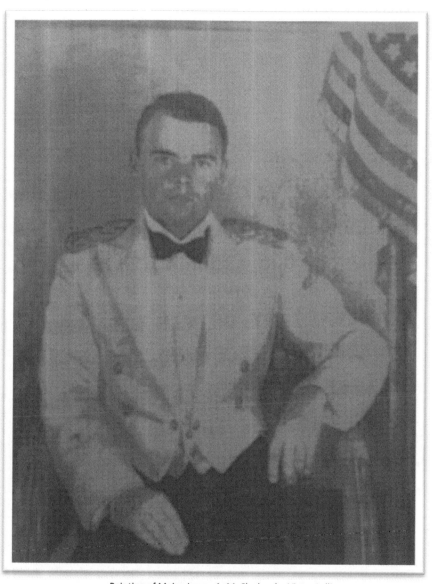

Painting of Major James A. McCloskey by Victor Lallier.
SOURCE: *U.S. Army McCloskey General Hospital, 1942-1946, Temple, Texas*, p. 11.

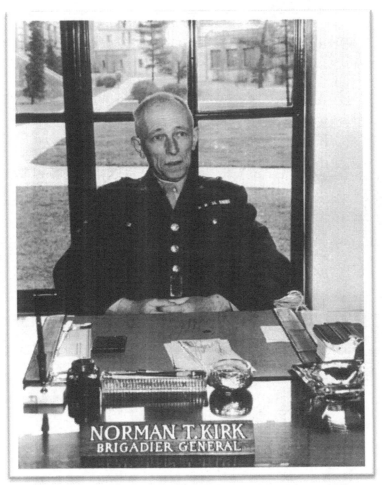

Brigadier General, Norman T. Kirk, Surgeon General of the U.S. Army, 1942.
SOURCE: Wikimedia Commons, public domain.

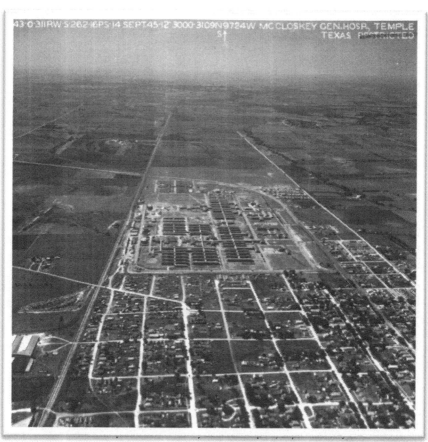

SOURCE: U.S. National Library of Medicine, public domain.

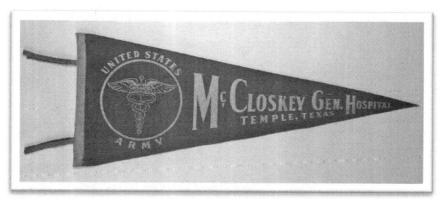

McCloskey General Hospital pennant. SOURCE: Collection of Denise Karimkhani.

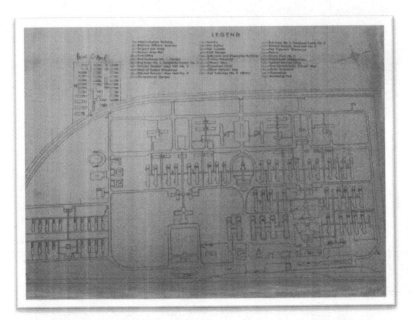

Map of McCloskey General Hospital showing Prisoner-of-War Camp. SOURCE: Olin E. Teague Veterans' Center Medical Library Archives.

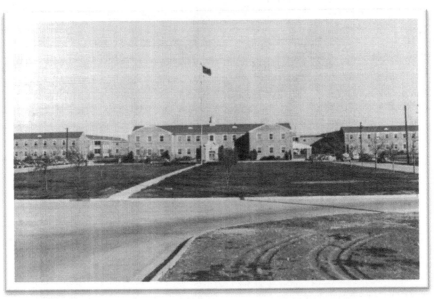

McCloskey General Hospital entrance and administration building. SOURCE: Collection of Sue Roeder Groveunder.

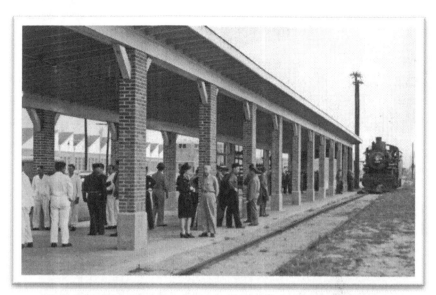

Staff at McCloskey General Hospital await the arrival of a hospital train, 1942.
Fred Springer Archives, Railroad and Heritage Museum. SOURCE: *Temple Daily
Telegram,* July 24, 2016.

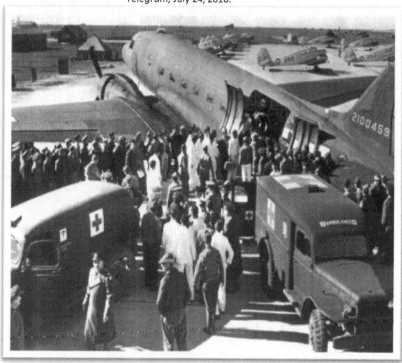

Army attendants help unload wounded soldiers from three planes in Temple in January
1944. SOURCE: Collection of Weldon Cannon and Patricia Benoit. *Temple Daily Telegram,*
January 7, 2019.

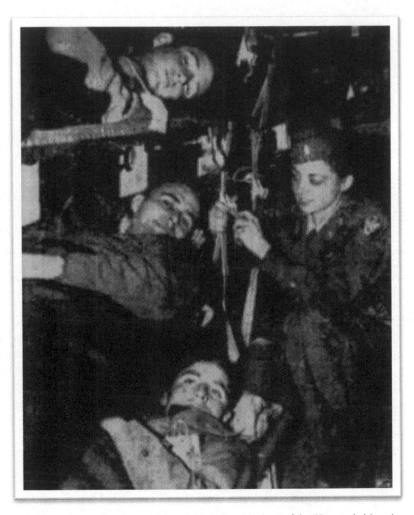

Lieut. M. A. D'Eletto, army nurse (R), makes comfortable three of the 75 wounded American war veterans who were flown to McCloskey General Hospital at Temple, Texas, from Charleston, S.C. The trio (top to bottom): Cpl. Jack G. White, Belton, Texas; Pfc. Jesse L. Stajanik, Temple, Texas; and Sgt. Boytt Impson, Durant, Okla. SOURCE: *Corsicana Daily Sun*, January 12, 1944, p. 10.

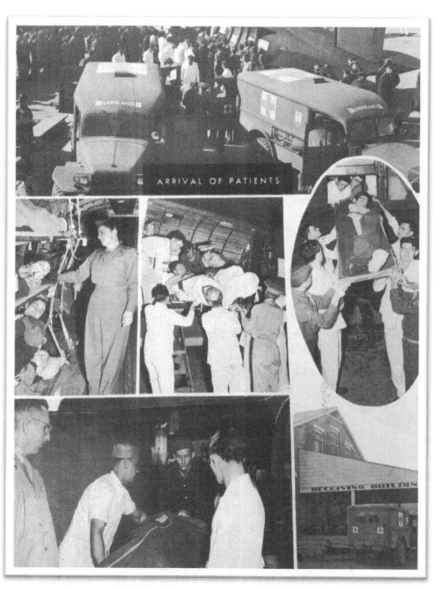

Arrival of patients at McCloskey General Hospital. SOURCE: *McCloskey General Hospital: Happiness, Kindness and Efficiency, Temple, Texas,* n.d.

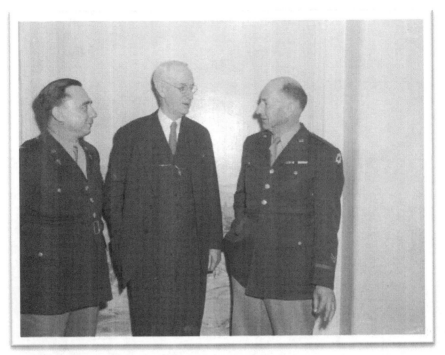

Army surgeons from McCloskey Hospital attend a symposium on reconstructive surgery at a meeting of the Texas Surgical Society at Hotel Texas in April 1945. Left to right are Col. H. J. Jaworski, Dr. A Singleton, and Brigadier General J. A. Bethea. SOURCE: Courtesy, *Fort Worth Star Telegram* Collection, Special Collections, The University of Texas at Arlington Libraries.

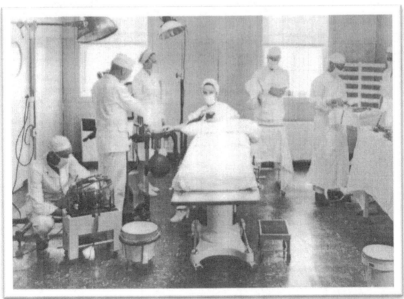

McCloskey General Hospital operating room. SOURCE: *Temple, Texas: The Hospital Center of the South,* n.d.

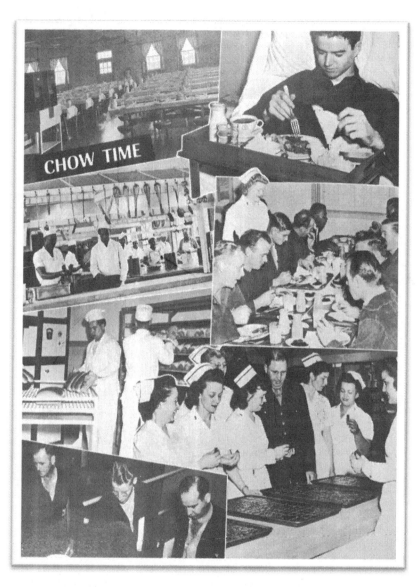

Dietetics at McCloskey General Hospital. SOURCE: *McCloskey General Hospital: Happiness, Kindness and Efficiency, Temple, Texas*, n.d.

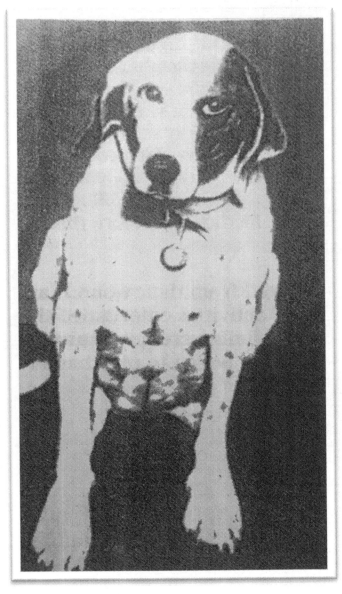

Maggie McCloskey, canine mascot. SOURCE: *U.S. Army McCloskey General Hospital, 1942-1946, Temple, Texas*, p. 32.

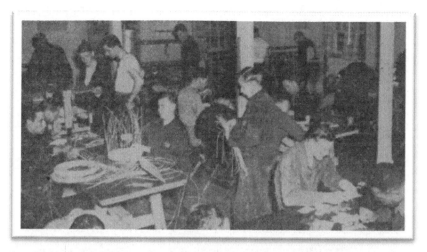

Beneficial in the rehabilitation of war wounded is this occupational therapy room at McCloskey General Hospital. Note the youth at center left busily engaged with basket-weaving. To his right is another operating a loom, while, at far right, another veteran is making a brightly-hued rug. SOURCE: Photograph by U.S. Army Signal Corps. *The Austin American-Statesman,* March 10, 1944, p. 15.

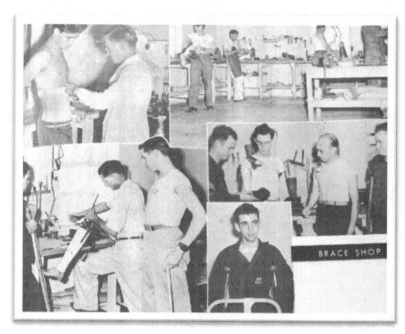

Brace shop at McCloskey General Hospital. SOURCE: *McCloskey General Hospital: Happiness, Kindness and Efficiency, Temple, Texas,* n.d.

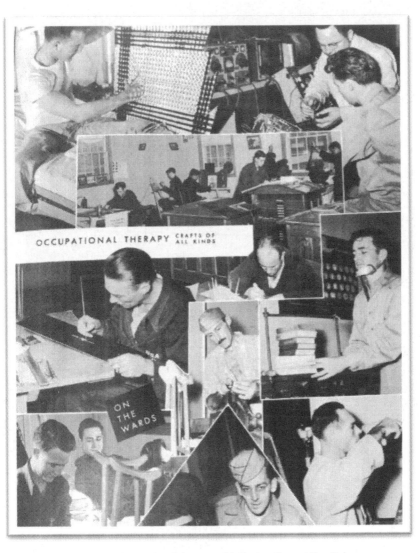

Occupational therapy at McCloskey General Hospital.
SOURCE: *McCloskey General Hospital: Happiness, Kindness and Efficiency, Temple, Texas*, n.d.

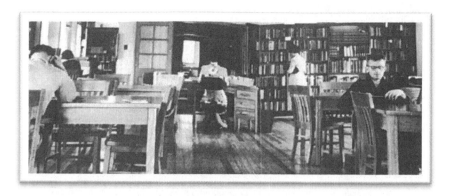

Library at McCloskey General Hospital.
SOURCE: *McCloskey General Hospital: Happiness, Kindness and Efficiency, Temple, Texas*, n.d.

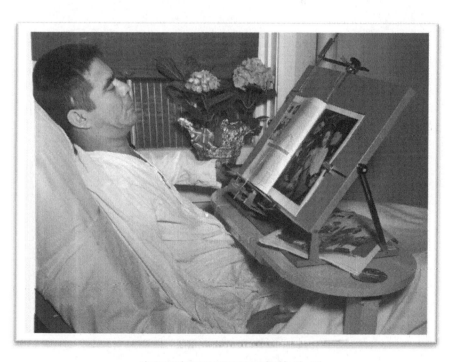

Automatic page turner supplied by the Library.
SOURCE: Olin E. Teague Veterans' Center Medical Library Archives.

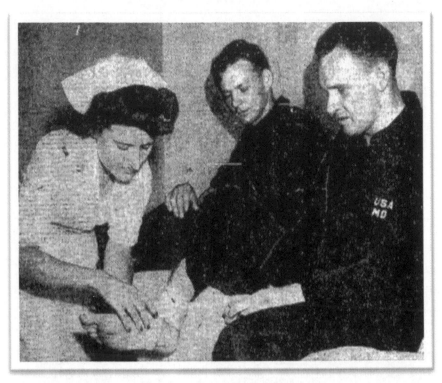

Sgt. Ralph O. Spence, (R) of Logan, Ohio, shot in the heel by a Jap woman sniper on Buna, gets his wound dressed by Lieut. Dorothy Loeffler, nurse at McCloskey hospital in Temple, Texas. Cpl. J. B. Capps of Jaking, Ga., waits for the nurse to dress his arm. He was wounded on Attu. SOURCE: *San Antonio Light*, July 8, 1943, p. 1

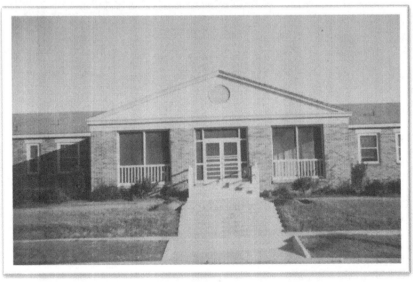

Nurses' quarters. SOURCE: Olin E. Teague Veterans' Center Medical Library Archives.

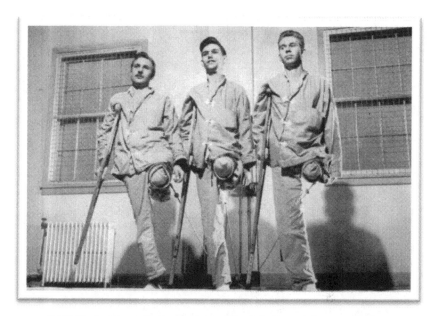

At U.S. Medical Corp's McCloskey General Hospital, three soldiers exercise the stumps of their left legs in preparation for the use of artificial limbs. SOURCE: *Life Magazine*, January 31, 1944, p. 69.

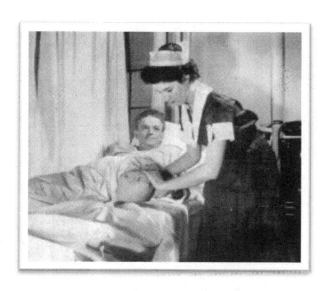

Stump is massaged by a physiotherapist. Massage is, in effect, a kind of passive exercise. It helps to restore blood circulation and build up muscle tone for the work of moving an artificial limb. SOURCE: *Life Magazine*, January 31, 1944, p. 69.

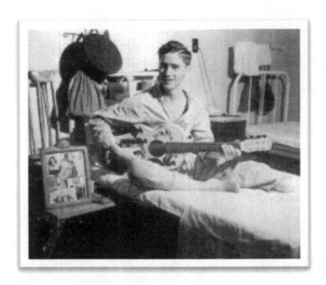

Private Tom Starr of Ballinger, Texas, lost his left leg following a shattering land-mine wound in Tunisia. The Army prepares soldiers psychologically for artificial limbs before the first fitting. SOURCE: *Life Magazine*, January 31, 1944, p. 69.

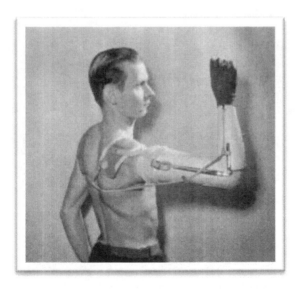

Artificial arm is made of plastic and metal to minimize its weight. To bend arm at elbow, soldier contract back muscles which pulls on leather thong attached to wrist. SOURCE: *Life Magazine*, January 31, 1944, p. 70.

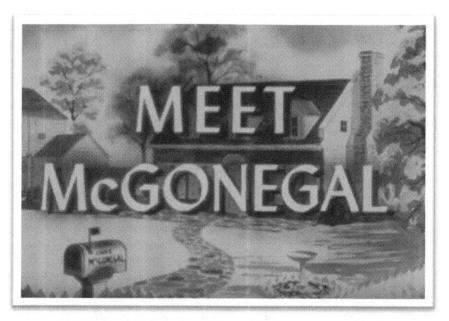

Meet McGonegal documentary film. Created by the Department of Defense,
Department of the Army. Office of the Chief Signal Officer, 1944. U.S. National Archives, 35836.
https://www.youtube.com/watch?v=FSLj5_HgYlo

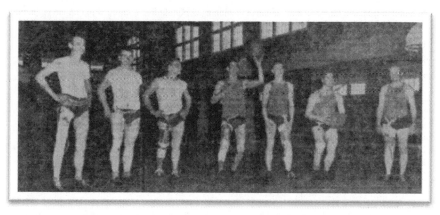

McCloskey's Purple Heart basketball team warms up in the general hospital's gym at Temple.
All members are leg amputees and battle casualties, but are still good shots--in fact, they
haven't lost a game this year. Left to right, they are: T-5 Charles S. Ramsey, Mansfield, La.; Capt.
Clyde T. Jetton, Salina, Okla.; T-Sgt. Allen S. Monts, Charleston, Ill.; Pfc. Pete A. Ochoa,
Galveston; Pfc. Erwin L. Moore, Caldwell; Pvt. Edward I Pace, Monticello, Ark., and T-5 Arvie
Walker, Lufkin. SOURCE: *The Austin American-Statesman*, February 26, 1946, p. 9.

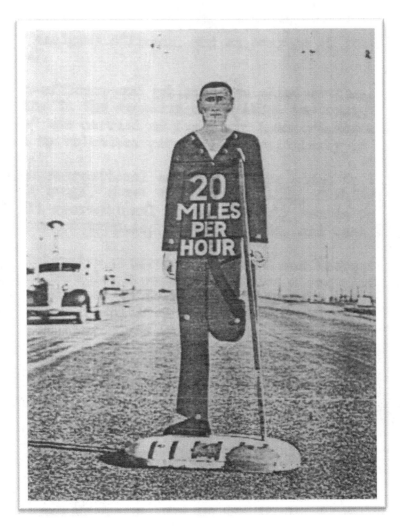

Traffic safety sign at McCloskey General Hospital.
SOURCE: James A. Bethea, "*Annual Report of McCloskey General Hospital, Temple, Texas For the Calendar Year 1945*" (Temple, TX: McCloskey General Hospital, January 1, 1946).

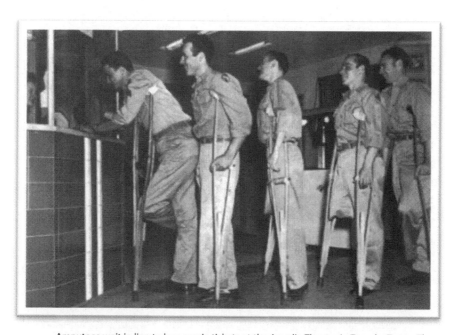

Amputees wait in line to buy movie tickets at the Arcadia Theater in Temple, Texas. The men (from left): Sgt. Joe Bone of Gadsden, Alabama; Pfc. Marvin Shaw of Van Buren, Arkansas; Pfc. William Warwick of Knoxville, Tennessee; Pfc. Ernest Petty of Dubuque, Iowa, and Pfc. Carl H. Fry of Wichita, Kansas. SOURCE: Collection of Weldon Cannon and Patricia Benoit.

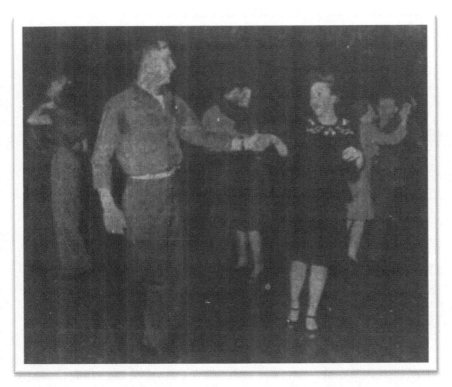

One-legged vet wins jitterbug contest. Pfc. Seb J. Wagner of New England, North Dakota, puts aside his crutches and with his partner, Lenora Durbin, Temple, Texas, literally "walked away" with first prize money and stopped the show with his dancing ability at a WAC "jitterbug contest" at McCloskey General Hospital, Temple, Texas. He is waiting for an artificial leg to replace his own lost in the Italian theatre. SOURCE: Signal Corps. Photo via NEA. SOURCE: *The Austin American-Statesman*, January 23, 1946, p. 7.

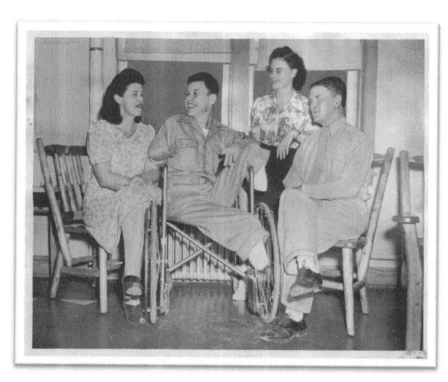

Sgt. Elmer Morris, Oklahoma war hero, shown with his mother, Mrs. E. L. Morris of Ringling, (L); his wife, Velma Lee, and his father, E. L. Morris, on a visit to McCloskey General Hospital in Temple, Texas. Photograph by U.S. Signal Corps. SOURCE: Courtesy, The Gateway to Oklahoma History.

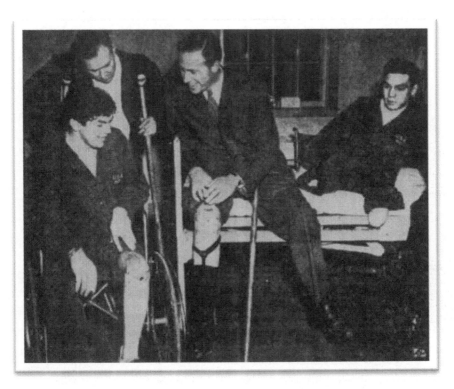

The Hon. Richard Wood (with cane), son of Lord & Lady Halifax, who paid a visit to Austin last week and addressed the house and senate, and Corp. George Foster (in wheelchair) of Orrville, Ohio, both of whom lost legs in action against the Germans, compared their new limbs at McCloskey General Hospital, Temple, Texas. Pvt. Clifford Warren (crutches) of Topeka, Kan., and Pvt. Ralph Rose (R) of Portsmouth, Ohio, look on. Wood lost both legs in North Africa. SOURCE: AP photo from Signal Corps. *The Austin American-Statesman*, March 22, 1945, p. 7.

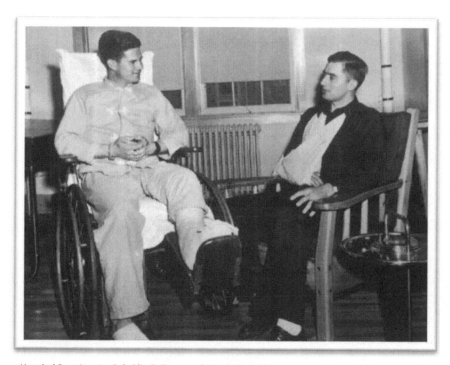

Hospital Reunion. Lt. Col. Olin E. Teague of Bryan, Texas (L) meets an officer of his command, Lt. Ither D. Malone of Waurika, Okla., at McCloskey General Hospital, Temple, Tex., where both are recovering from wounds received in action. SOURCE: Olin E. Teague Veterans' Center Medical Library Archives.

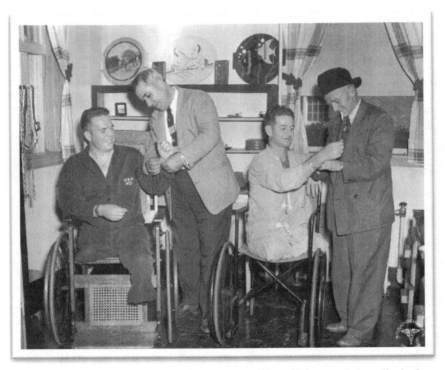

At McCloskey General Hospital, Temple, Texas, two soldiers with leg amputations, Charles R. Rummell (L) and Warren C. Cowen, receive silver ID bracelets from Houston businessmen Andrew Vassiliades (L) and Andy Anderson in November 1944. [Public domain photograph by U.S. Army Signal Corps]. Courtesy, Warren C. Cowen Papers, Special Collections, The University of Texas at Arlington Libraries.

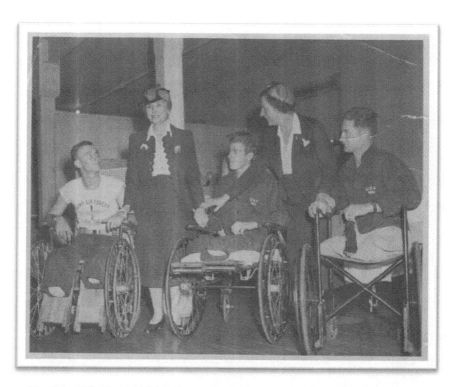

Miss Helen Keller (L, standing) and her companion, Miss Polly Thompson (R, standing), talking with World War II veterans at McCloskey General Hospital. Pictured sitting in their wheelchairs are, left to right, Corporal Abe C. Beal, of Springfield, Missouri, Private Douglass F. Megehee, of Ardmore, Oklahoma, and Sergeant Warren Cowen; 11/24/1944. [Public domain photograph by U.S. Army Signal Corps]. Courtesy, *Warren C. Cowen Papers*, Special Collections, The University of Texas at Arlington Libraries.

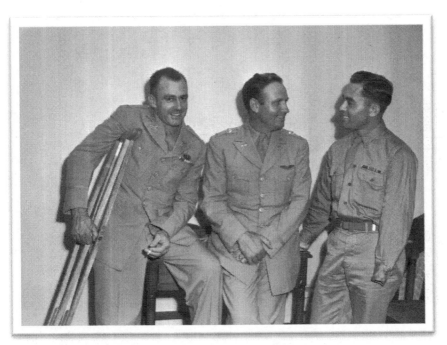

The Singing Cowboy Gene Autry is visiting wounded war veterans at McCloskey General Hospital in 1944. He is pictured with two veterans. From left to right, are Lieutenant (Lt.) Ralph S. McGill, paratrooper; Technical Sergeant Gene Autry, and Corporal (Cpl.) Woodrow Brown. Courtesy, *Fort Worth Star-Telegram* Collection, Special Collections, The University of Texas at Arlington Libraries.

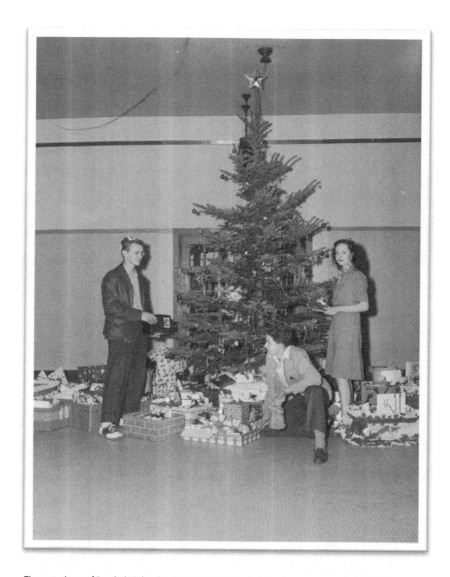

Three students of Paschal High School are transferring gifts from home rooms and placing them under the school Christmas tree in 1944. The students are, left to right, Clark Gillespie, Odin Wilson, and Mary McKinney. The gifts will be delivered to wounded servicemen at McCloskey General Hospital, Waco Army Air Field, and Camps Perrin and Wolters. Courtesy, *Fort Worth Star-Telegram* Collection, Special Collections, The University of Texas at Arlington Libraries.

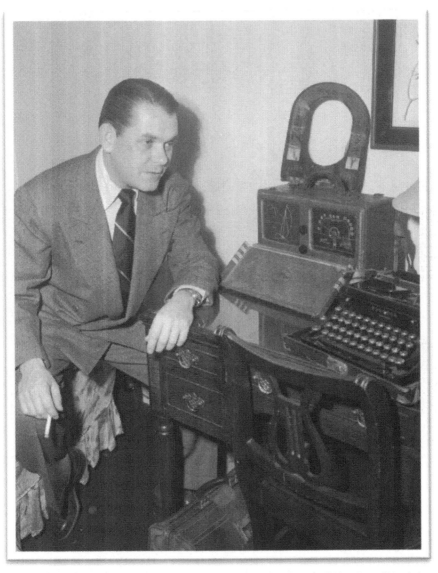

Frankie Masters and his band appeared for the Coca-Cola broadcast from McCloskey General Hospital and will play a similar program for the men stationed at Love Field. Courtesy, *Fort Worth Star-Telegram* Collection, Special Collections, The University of Texas at Arlington Libraries.

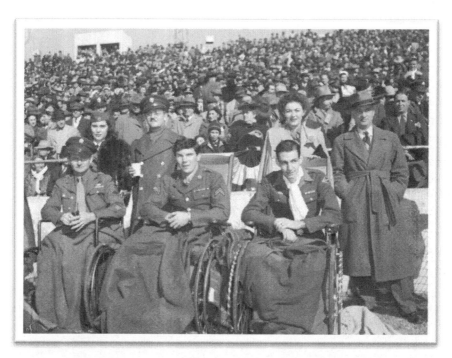

Cotton Bowl Game spectators on New Year's Day 1945. Left to right, Staff Sergeant Warren Cowen, Corporal George Foster and Private First-Class Martin Gubanowich, McCloskey veterans. Standing behind them are, left to right, Miss Jimmie Ruth Cheatham, Sergeant Eddie Payne and Miss Pennie Logan of Oklahoma City. Courtesy, *Fort Worth Star-Telegram* Collection, Special Collections, The University of Texas at Arlington Libraries.

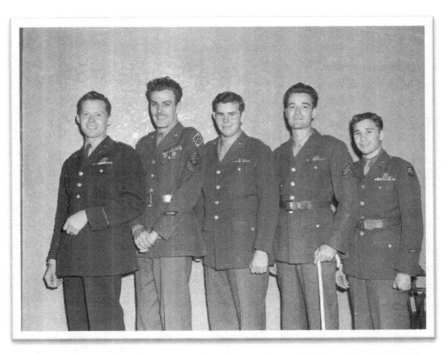

Wounded veterans from McCloskey General Hospital are volunteers in the Fourth War Loan Drive in 1944. They are, left to right, Lieutenant Cullen E. Cole, Sergeant Harry J. Banan, Private Robert Thad Knittel, Corporal Lee W. McBride and Private First-Class Thomas F. McNeely. All five men wear the Purple Heart. They are lending their help to "back the attack" in Fort Worth's Fourth War Loan campaign. Courtesy, *Fort Worth Star-Telegram* Collection, Special Collections, The University of Texas at Arlington Libraries.

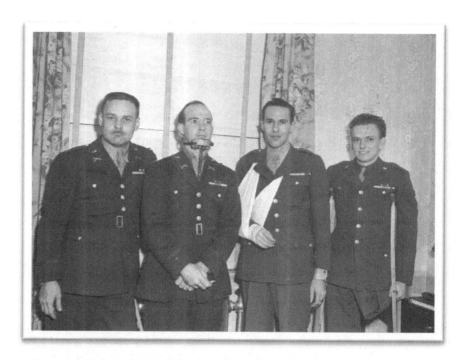

Four wounded veterans from McCloskey General Hospital are volunteers in the Fourth War Loan Drive in January 1944. They are, left to right, Captain Joseph E. Southworth, Captain David C. Kelly Junior, Private First-Class Hugh E. Rueter, and Private First-Class Hershel T. Calhoun. Courtesy, *Fort Worth Star-Telegram* Collection, Special Collections, The University of Texas at Arlington Libraries.

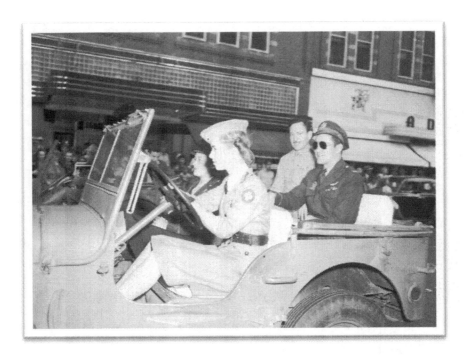

Victory Loan Drive. Major John B. Smith and Lieutenant Sam Rubenstein (wearing dark glasses), both wounded veterans from McCloskey General Hospital in Temple, are driven by Miss Maxine Middleton of the Red Cross Motor Corps in October 1945. Courtesy, *Fort Worth Star-Telegram* Collection, Special Collections, The University of Texas at Arlington Libraries.

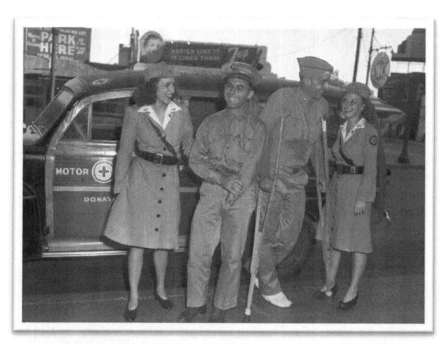

American Red Cross Motor Corps volunteers are driving two wounded veterans from Temple, Texas to Fort Worth to give a speech at the bond premiere in July 1944. The volunteers and veterans left to right, are Miss Frances Nelson, Corporal Woodrow Brown, Lieutenant Ralph S. McGill, and Miss Doris Jean Bridges. Courtesy, *Fort Worth Star-Telegram* Collection, Special Collections, The University of Texas at Arlington Libraries.

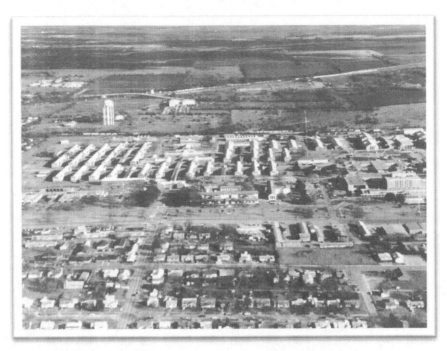

Aerial view of McCloskey Veterans Hospital. Color photo, year unknown.
SOURCE: Olin E. Teague Veterans' Center Medical Library Archives.

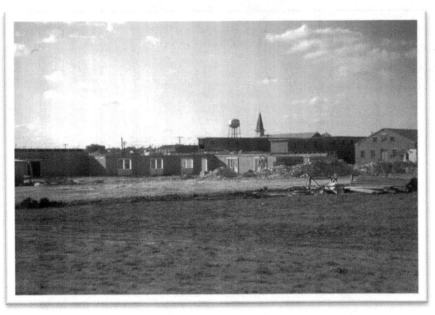

Construction of the new veterans' hospital. Color slide by Helen R. Woolley, ca. 1965-1966.
SOURCE: Personal photos of Denise Karimkhani.

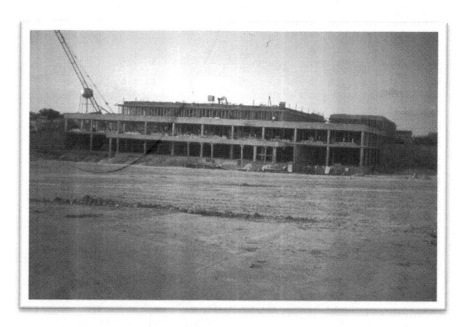

Construction of the new veterans' hospital. Color slide by Helen R. Woolley, ca. 1965-1966.
SOURCE: Personal photos of Denise Karimkhani.

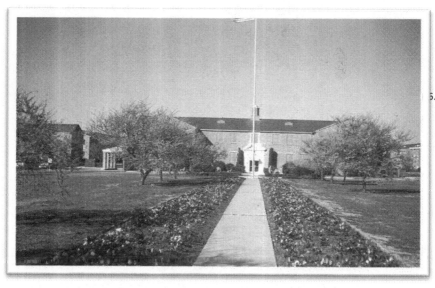

McCloskey Veterans Hospital Administration Building. Color slide by Helen R. Woolley, year
unknown. SOURCE: Personal photos of Denise Karimkhani.

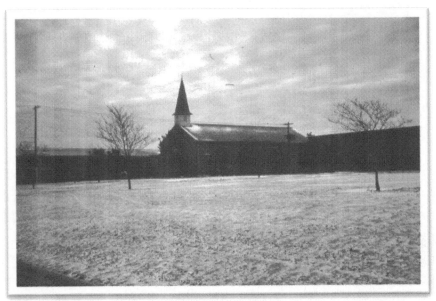

McCloskey chapel in the snow. Color slide by Helen R. Woolley, year unknown.
Personal photos of Denise Karimkhani.

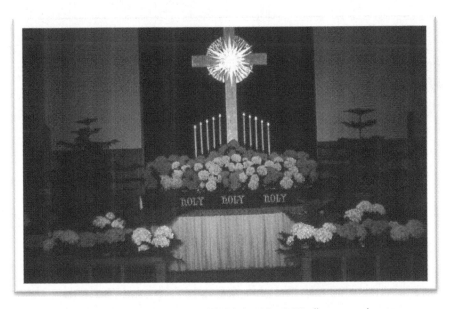

Chapel decorated for Christmas. Color slide by Helen R. Woolley, year unknown.
SOURCE: Personal photos of Denise Karimkhani.

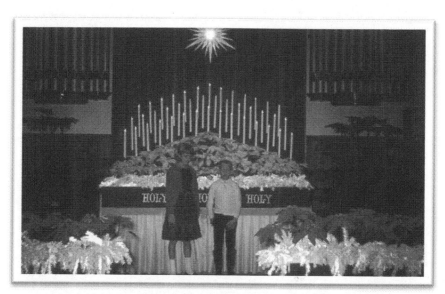

Denise & Kyle Woolley in the chapel. Color slide by Helen R. Woolley, ca. 1965.
SOURCE: Personal photos of Denise Karimkhani.

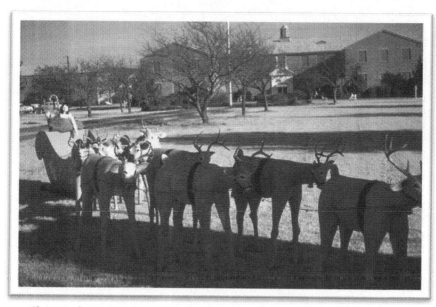

Christmas decorations on the hospital grounds. Color slide by Helen R. Woolley, year unknown.
SOURCE: Personal photos of Denise Karimkhani.

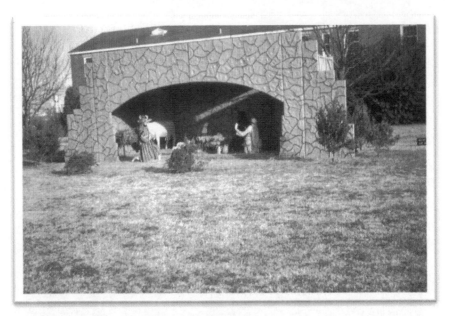

Christmas decorations on the hospital grounds. Color slide by Helen R. Woolley, year unknown.
SOURCE: Personal photos of Denise Karimkhani.

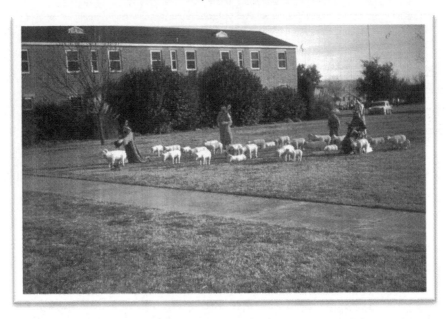

Christmas decorations on the hospital grounds. Color slide by Helen R. Woolley, year unknown.
SOURCE: Personal photos of Denise Karimkhani.

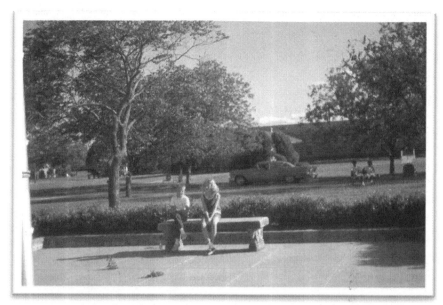

Kyle & Denise Woolley in front of Administration Building. Color slide by Helen R. Woolley, ca. 1965. SOURCE: Personal photos of Denise Karimkhani.

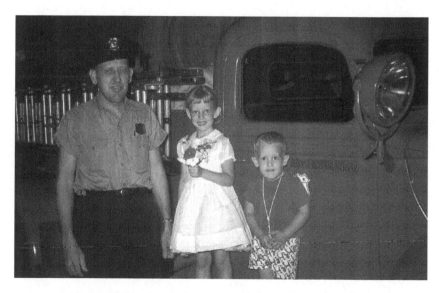

Aubrey Woolley, Denise & Kyle at McCloskey fire station. Color slide by Helen R. Woolley, ca. 1959. SOURCE: Personal photos of Denise Karimkhani.

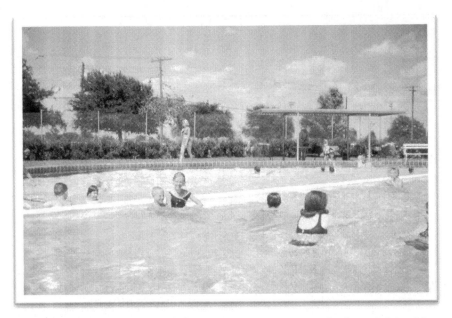

McCloskey Veterans Hospital swimming pool with Kyle & Denise Woolley (center). Color slide by Helen R. Woolley, ca. 1965. SOURCE: Personal photos of Denise Karimkhani.

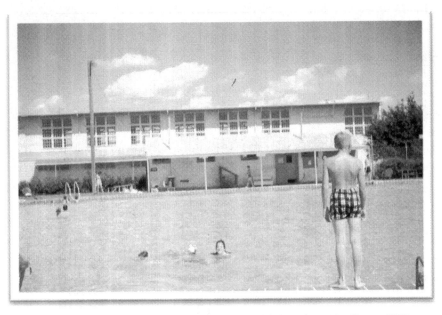

McCloskey Veterans Hospital swimming pool. Color slide by Helen R. Woolley, ca. 1965. SOURCE: Personal photos of Denise Karimkhani.

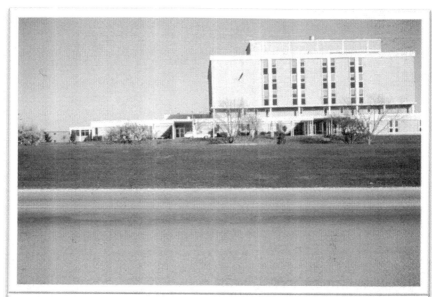

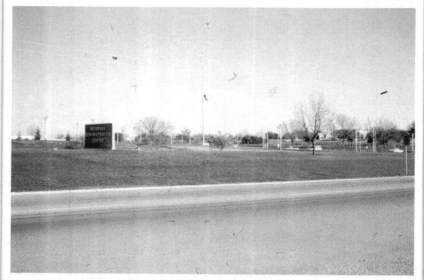

Veterans Administration Center. Color slides by Helen R. Woolley, year unknown. SOURCE:
Personal photos of Denise Karimkhani.

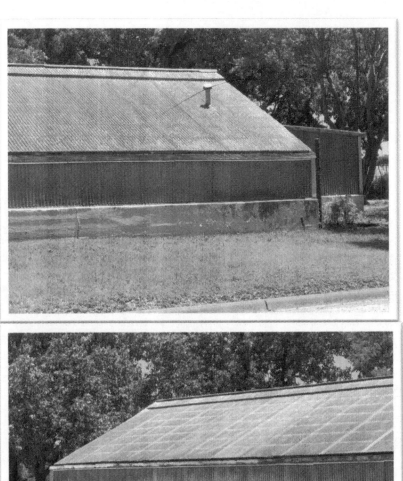

Greenhouse funded by Rotarians and built by P.O.W. labor still standing, 2019. Digital photos by Denise Karimkhani.

Chapter 7: Behind the Scenes

Early ambulation and use of elastic stockings were not the only new ideas developed during the war. According to Colonel Jaworski, significant strides were made in surgical procedures and anesthesia. He said, "I believe that one of the greatest advantages, or rather greatest improvements in anesthesia were developed during the war in closed endotracheal type of anesthesia especially. We were able to operate on pulmonary conditions, on chest injuries, under closed types of anesthesia which were hardly heard of before World War II."[216]

Jaworski further told of his experiences with studying the use of penicillin. McCloskey was one of the hospitals designated by the Surgeon General to experiment with the drug which arrived under the protection of an armored car. Jaworski said,

> I remember so well that we started with very small doses, maybe five or ten units. Then, of course, we began to study bigger doses and bigger doses. We had to be extremely careful for reactions. We had to carry the antidote with us to use in case of a reaction and carefully instruct all doctors in its use and how to prevent reactions, and, if they did occur, how to treat them.[217]

Alexander Fleming discovered penicillin in 1928 in England, but he soon found that penicillin was difficult to produce in large quantities. He continued to work with penicillin for another twelve years and his research paved the way for the work of Howard Florey, Ernst Chain, and Norman Heatley at Oxford University. On May 25, 1939, the scientists conducted an experiment using two groups of mice, one group injected with *Streptococcus* and penicillin and one group left untreated. By the next day, the control mice all died; the treated mice were still alive. The researchers published their findings in *The Lancet* in August 1940. The Oxford team worked to purify the drug and began to test its clinical effectiveness on humans. In February 1941, the first person to receive penicillin was an Oxford policeman with a serious infection throughout his body. The administration of penicillin resulted in dramatic improvement in his condition within 24 hours. Unfortunately, the limited supply was depleted, and the policeman later died. Other patients received the drug with great success, and the scientists published their findings. Because of wartime commitments and the fear of German invasion, the British government was unable to provide funding for medical research or mass production of penicillin, so Florey and Heatley turned to the United States for assistance. In 1941, the supply of penicillin in the United States was not enough to treat even a single patient; in December 1941, the U.S. entered the war and the need for penicillin became urgent. The U.S. government dedicated substantial resources to its mass production, and by September 1943, the levels were high enough to satisfy the demands of the Allied Armed Forces and the plans for the invasion of Europe. Overseas shipments of penicillin commenced, and by October, penicillin was a standard therapeutic item.

Earlier in the year, the army selected ten general hospitals to investigate the use of penicillin in the treatment of surgical infection. McCloskey received its first shipment in July 1943.[218] Bushnell and Halloran General Hospitals were designated teaching centers where medical officers from other general hospitals were trained in penicillin studies. "Penicillin committees" were established in hospitals to evaluate the cases in which the still scarce drug should be used. Colonel Jaworski emphasized, "It is available only in small quantities, and the men who use it are trained for that purpose at Bushnell General Hospital in Utah before being allowed to take it up."[219] Penicillin injections were first administered at McCloskey to a group of six seriously wounded soldiers with blood infections who miraculously survived. Major George F. Wollgast, a McCloskey orthopedist, reported on this and other uses of the drug including treatment of gonorrhea, meningitis, bone infections, and pneumonia. Once the use of penicillin was authorized at McCloskey, 613 cases were treated during the year 1944 according to General Bethea who wrote, "Penicillin has been used judiciously and effectively with resultant decrease in morbidity, operative delay, and disability, which usually are associated with prolonged infections."[220]

On December 13, 1943, in a program broadcast over WOR, Major General Norman T. Kirk told the American Pharmaceutical Manufacturers' Association that as the Army Surgeon General "it is with great pride that I am able to report today to the fathers, mothers, wives and sweethearts of our fighting men that penicillin is literally in mass production" and that it would be available in "adequate supplies for military and civilian needs within the next six months." [221] Kirk hailed the drug as one of the "three heroes of World War 2" with the other two being blood plasma and the mobility and organization of the medical services which ensured prompt and efficient treatment. Major General Kirk assured the public that "the wounded soldier in this global war, though he is exposed to almost every health hazard known to man, still has a better chance of surviving and returning safely home than ever before." [222] A month earlier, the first penicillin known to be released for emergency civilian use was flown to West Texas from McCloskey hospital to treat a gas gangrene infection threatening the life of a 13-year-old Abilene youth, Wayne Haynes. The 500,000 units were transported by airman Jack Hughes on the approval of Dr. Chester Keefer at Evans Memorial Hospital in Boston. By January 1944, twenty-eight general hospitals were engaged in penicillin studies related to surgical infections. Penicillin proved to be effective in treating wound infections and was an important factor in reducing hospital stays as well as mortality rates. With the increased production of penicillin in 1944 and 1945, restrictions on its use were lifted, and by March 1945, nearly all demands were met. [223]

In December 1944, McCloskey General Hospital was designated as a plastic eye center, administered by a specially trained dental officer. In 1945, officials at McCloskey broke army secrecy to reveal the details about the development of a new plastic eye. For generations, Germany held a monopoly on the production of artificial glass eyes, and in 1933, prohibited the export of raw materials including the special glass from which the eyes were made. Those who needed glass eyes were unable to obtain them. A story in *The Milwaukee Journal*, April 26, 1945, reported that three army dentists (Captain Stanley F. Erpf, Major Milton S. Wirtz, and Major Victor H. Dietz) discovered the secret of lifelike plastic eyes. Using an alginate plastic mixed with water to make a paste, the expert made an impression of the patient's eye socket. It was used at body temperature and caused no pain or discomfort. The patient's exact measurements were taken. The impression was used to make a wax model, and from it a plaster replica. Veins made of fibers of red rayon were added to simulate the patient's natural eye. The final step involved dipping the eye into a clear solution of the plastic and holding it in the air to dry. This gave the finished eye a gleaming fluid coating like the liquid that covers the normal eye in real life. Major R. A. Mitchell, chief of the artificial eye laboratory at McCloskey, stated that the new plastic eyes last a lifetime, were unbreakable, and defied detection. General James Bethea said that he and most nurses were unable to discern the difference between a plastic and a real eye. An Austin man, Technical Sergeant William S. Falkenbury, was the recipient of the first plastic eye made in the McCloskey laboratory.[224] With pride Major Mitchell told the story of Lieutenant Wayland Swain of Dalton, Georgia, who was blinded by an explosion of a land mine in Europe. A pair of medium blue eyes was made for Swain whose wife said they were identical to his real eyes. The plastic eye was lightweight and moved naturally with the real eye. As Mitchell put it, "We've whipped the Germans again—at their own game."[225]

Despite the positive outcomes, McCloskey became the focus of national attention after a negative story circulated in the Hearst newspapers regarding the treatment of one particular eye patient, Robert Wetzel of McCloud, California. Wetzel was wounded in Italy and lost sight in one eye. According to the press, Wetzel was discharged from McCloskey after "receiving improper care and was even forced to pay for his own glasses."[226] A subsequent investigation was conducted by Gordon Fulcher, editor of the *Austin American-Statesman*, who personally visited the hospital and published his findings:

> The Hearst writers would have the public believe that the boy was turned out and forced to buy his own glasses. The facts are that the boy was given the best medical science has to offer in his treatment. He was given a prescription, before being discharged from the hospital for glasses to replace those already given him by the government. The new glasses were not supposed to have been worn until his eye had strengthened sufficiently to wear them. Instead the boy bought glasses on the new prescription from the McCloskey PX before leaving. On his arrival home the Hearst papers circulated stories that the boy was forced to buy his own glasses. Had he waited until the proper time for him to wear the new glasses he would have been furnished them by the Veterans Administration in his own state...

Representatives of the *Statesman* randomly interviewed wounded soldiers at McCloskey and received "nothing but the highest praise of the treatment they received from hospital authorities and workers." J.M. Walker, aide-de-camp of the Veterans of Foreign Wars, who interviewed more than 1,000 men at McCloskey for membership in the V.F.W. reported that he had "yet to get one complaint from the boys about the treatment they get at the hospital." When Lieutenant Paul A. Farrell, a former Hearst newspaperman and patient at McCloskey, read the story in the February 13, 1944, edition of the *San Antonio Light*, he immediately wrote a letter to the editor, denying the Hearst story and vindicating the hospital staff:

131

I think I can speak for the majority if not all of those men—officers and enlisted men   alike—and they include groups from the air corps, ordnance, artillery, infantry, tank corps, quartermaster, etc., in that they have the highest praise for the medical officers of this hospital; for their treatment, their kindness, their courtesy and general interest in the welfare of all patients. Also, the nurses of this institution as well as the ward men and office help can be included when there are any expressions of patients' gratitude to be handed out. [227]

McCloskey doctors clarified the details of the Wetzel case. Wetzel was fitted with glasses at Stark General Hospital in South Carolina before being transferred to Temple. At McCloskey he was fitted with an artificial eye for his left eye. The foreign particles in his right eye were not treated since that was his only remaining vision. McCloskey officials stated that Wetzel simply misunderstood the medical instructions he received, and they believe he did not mean to indict anyone at the hospital. General Bethea sent a refund check of eight dollars to Wetzel and declared that the soldier had misunderstood directions. Bethea's letter said in part:

We knew nothing about any of this until we read it in the paper. We have certainly made a hard and conscientious effort to see that all of our patients get the best care possible while they are here. Incidentally Colonel Smith is not only one of the leading eye specialists of the country, professor of eye diseases at one of our leading universities, but he is one of the kindest hearted men I have ever known, and it grieves him to think that you were not satisfied. He does not believe that the glasses you   ordered   will   be satisfactory at the present time but believes they will be after you have accustomed your eyes to the glasses you had upon leaving here, which will take a few months. [228]

Another negative report surfaced in 1944 when the *San Francisco Examiner* told of Lawrence Edward Mahoney of New York who with "hands gone, blind, deaf, boy left to shift for himself by Army." Stationed at Camp Hood, Mahoney was injured by a defective grenade that blew off his hands, destroyed his left eye, and ruptured both ear drums. Mahoney described his four months at McCloskey:

> It was pretty grim. Nobody came in to help you, to tell you how to use your new hands. You just lay in bed all day. Sometimes, because the blocks hurt and I'd have them off, an orderly would come through, take them off the windowsill, and throw them on the bed, 'Put your hands on,' he'd say. So I'd put them on. [229]

Mahoney said that he left McCloskey with $132 in back pay and railroad fare for the trip home, but never received any rehabilitation while there. The story was neither confirmed nor denied by McCloskey officials. The newspaper stated that his story was featured to highlight the "experience of thousands of neglected veterans like Lawrence Edward Mahoney, many of them in even more desperate circumstances" for whom the Hearst newspapers sought justice. Throughout the war, erroneous newspaper stories circulated concerning so-called "basket cases" recuperating in general hospitals. These were men who had lost both arms and both legs and supposedly had to be transported in a basket rather than on a stretcher. *Time Magazine* reported on the first U.S. "basket case" of World War II, Master Sergeant Frederic Hensel of Corbin, Kentucky. [230] Hensel stepped on a mine in Okinawa, and the explosion blew off both legs above the knee, his left arm above the elbow, and badly mangled his right hand. It was also reported that many unidentified patients languished in hospitals. Captain Moss, McCloskey public relations officer, appealed to newspaper editors to dispel such rumors, saying neither class of patient existed in any of the 63 general hospitals. Personal identification records were thorough and complete.

In contrast to the occasional unfavorable and generally unwarranted negative publicity, General Bethea often received and sometimes published warm, enthusiastic letters from discharged patients like the one below:

Dear Sir,
May I be permitted this liberty to express to you, sir, and through you, to the entire ward organization of Ward 117A my most sincere gratitude for the excellent care and treatment accorded me during my convalescence here these many weeks. Upon the eve of my departure to a veteran's hospital in the northland, I reflect with genuine gratification upon the untiring kindness, and watchful care of this ward staff not only in my case but also in the case of many soldiers receiving care and treatment in this ward. It is an assuring, comforting thought to a soldier to know that whatever the illness or wound may be there is provided for him the very best in medical attention and care at the army's general hospitals staffed by the most skillful of officers representing the medical profession assisted by a most highly and efficiently trained personnel. God grant that each and every soldier sent here to you and your staff for medical attention and treatment may leave this hospital with the same genuine feeling of gratitude and admiration that I take along with me as a cherished remembrance

of my stay here and of the very good efforts of Captain DeBold and his ward organization.
Thank you.
Respectfully submitted,
/s/ Pvt. A..... H.....
Ward 117 A[231]

The war wounded also benefited from the use of a long-neglected "magic metal" that aided in the repair and restoration of damaged nerves and shattered skulls. Tantalum was known to chemists, but its first wartime use was reported in 1940 by Canadian surgeon, Gerald L. Burke, who experimented with tantalum and found it useful for surgery. He stated in the *Canadian Medical Association Journal*, "To summarize its virtues: it is uniquely resistant to corrosion, is as strong as steel, and can be stamped, machined and drawn into wire. [232] McCloskey was one of sixteen hospitals designated as neuro-surgical centers where surgeries on the brain, spinal cord, and peripheral nerves were performed. Major William T. Haverfield, chief of the neuro-surgical division at McCloskey, used tantalum wire to join nerves severed by shellfire and embedded ultra-thin sheets of tantalum into the shattered skulls or abdominal walls of wounded soldiers.[233] Tantalum wire sutures, only one-fourth the diameter of a human hair, linked severed nerves, and restored normal motion. Major Haverfield explained that "the body receives it very well, better than any other foreign material." There are no reactions or irritations of the body tissues. Tantalum is soft and malleable and able to be drawn, cut, hammered and fitted into a plate right at the operating table. He went on to explain the procedure for filling in a bullet hole in a patient's skull:

> The scalp overlying the defect is turned down in a broad flap to expose the margins of the hole in the bone. X-ray film is used to make a pattern of this defect. When the film has been cut to fit the hole, it is then placed upon a thin sheet of

tantalum and the tantalum is cut around its margins. The piece of tantalum thus cut is next shaped to conform to the curvature of the skull in the region of the defect. When it has been shaped and fitted into the defect to replace the bone that has been lost, it is then wired into the margins of the defect with tantalum wire. The scalp is then placed back over this tantalum plate and sewed in place.

In 1944, one McCloskey dental officer was sent to the Tantalum Defense Corporation in Chicago for instruction on forming tantalum skull plates.[234] Once trained, the Dental Service constructed 45 plates for both the neurosurgical and plastic surgical branches. Dentists worked to continually improve and devise new methods so that all types and sizes of tantalum plate restorations were made at McCloskey. Tantalum continued to be used successfully for general surgery and neurosurgery implants with no problems reported in biocompatibility.

As an amputation center, McCloskey had the opportunity to try new and experimental procedures on patients. Overseas, some patients received emergency "guillotine" amputations, removing only so much of the hand or foot as was necessary to save the soldier's life and prevent the spread of infection. A final amputation was performed upon arrival back in the states. McCloskey surgeons often removed more of the arm or leg in the final amputation. When amputations were taking place, it was not uncommon for the nerve surgeon to schedule an adjacent operating room and at the same time obtain a short length of nerve cord from the amputation and suture it immediately while it was still alive to the nerve channel of his own patient. The first surgery of this type was performed at McCloskey in 1943. The doctor knew the patient would never have use of his arm so if the surgery proved successful and the nerve fibrils grew through the double suture of the cord splice, the surgeon would achieve a miracle of restoration. It was said that nerves grew at the rate of approximately an inch per month and by providing a channel for their growth, they would eventually reach their terminal again and successfully transmit the brain's messages to a limp hand or foot. In 1945, a new method of electrodiagnosis of peripheral nerve lesions was instituted at McCloskey but was too early in its use to be effectively evaluated and reported.

In 1945, McCloskey implemented a regimen of physical therapy using heavy resistance exercise with "striking success." Developed at Gardiner General Army Hospital in Chicago by Dr. Thomas Lanier DeLorme, the program used "iron boots" and pulleys and produced almost miraculous results. The methods helped patients recuperate more quickly and many regained full use of their legs. By speeding up rehabilitation, patient backlogs were reduced. As his methods evolved, Dr. DeLorme changed the terminology of his system to "Progressive Resistance Exercise" and continued to promote weight training throughout his career.[235]

Overall, wounded soldiers in the war had an excellent chance of recovery and resumption of normal life upon discharge from the hospital. The Office of War Information produced a poster entitled *Saving the Wounded* showing the improvement in lives saved between World War I and World War II. [236]

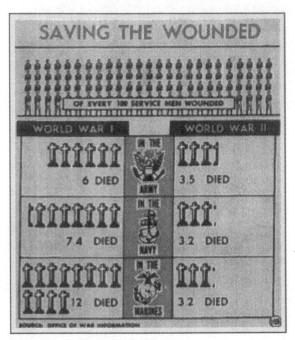

SOURCES: Maisel, 1944, back dust cover.

In 1944, it was reported that not only was the death rate from disease in the army lower than it was in World War I, but it was lower than the annual death rate in the army during any one of the previous ten years of peace.[237]

Chapter 8: Hearts Open, Sleeves Up

In early 1942, *New York Times* military editor Hanson Baldwin believed Americans needed a wake-up call to the grim realization that "this is a war we can lose" following American and British defeats in Europe and the Pacific.[238] He regularly used his newspaper column as a forum to shock reluctant, complacent citizens into the necessity of making greater sacrifices in order to win the war. As the general hospitals became populated with war wounded and the terrors of battle became all-too-real, donations of all sorts poured in from the grateful citizenry. The patients at McCloskey were living proof that Americans were willing to sacrifice and give generously to provide gifts of various kinds. Cheer funds were common, and the money collected was used to pay for soldiers' phone calls home, birthday parties, books, and other items to lift the spirits of wounded veterans. The Luther League of Peace Lutheran Church in Rockdale sponsored a cheer fund for McCloskey vets. Milk bottles were placed in businesses and a special Youth Service was held to take collections. The McCloskey Cheer Fund of Texas, started by Dick Freeman, sports editor of the *Houston Chronicle*, collected over $70,000. In 1948, $4,000 remained in the fund which Freeman then sent to McCloskey to pay for a Crouse-Hinds floodlight system for the baseball-softball field.[239]

Holidays were special times and donations came from service clubs, churches, Sunday School classes, and Christmas programs. On Thanksgiving evening in 1944, a benefit dance was held at SPJST Lodge Jaromir No. 54 in West, and $206.75 was donated to purchase Christmas gifts for McCloskey patients. In attendance at the dance were McCloskey patients and/or members of the staff including Sergeant Leo Schroeder, Sergeant Joe Foit, Private First Class Louis Gajdusek, Private Wick Devers, Private George E. Odem, and Sergeant Puckett "[240] A story in *The Nebraska State Journal* further demonstrated the generosity of the American people as they played Santa Claus to the men of Texas' 36th Division and Oklahoma's 45th Division who were wounded at Salerno.[241] For those patients who could only be home for Christmas in their dreams, Girl Scouts from Duluth, Minnesota, made 3,500 miniature tray favors, created from tiny birch logs, red candles and embellished with red bows. All McCloskey mess halls were adorned with Christmas trees, while the walls, windows and tables were festooned with red, white, and green decorations. A special Christmas dinner consisting of grapefruit-pineapple cocktail, roast turkey with sage dressing and giblet gravy, cranberry-orange relish, mashed potatoes, green beans, tomato stuffed with apple and celery, Parker House rolls, eggnog ice cream, fruit cake, candies, fruit, nuts, and coffee was planned by the hospital dietitians.

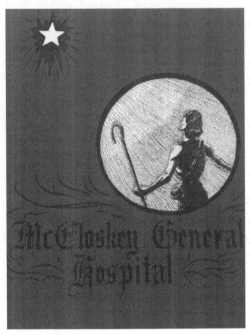

Christmas Menu and Employee Roster, 1944. SOURCE: Collection of Denise Karimkhani.

Organizations from New York, Ohio, Oklahoma, Nebraska, New Mexico, Texas, and other states sent more than 20,000 blocks of gifts.[242] Two McCloskey buildings housed Telephone Centers where operators on duty assisted patients with their calls daily and especially on holidays. One "special equipment" phone booth was large enough to allow boys in wheelchairs to have privacy while talking on the phone. For those patients who were confined to bed or did not have use of their arms, special headsets were provided, and amplifying telephones were available for patients with impaired hearing. Home-made goodies were discouraged by dietitians for fear of upsetting special diets. That did not deter Catholic women from Cameron sending "the largest cookie jar" containing 4,180 cookies to the men at McCloskey. [243] In lieu of cookies and candy, Austin citizens raised money for cigarettes. *The Austin American-Statesman* reported that the McCloskey cigarette fund had become the talk of the town with citizens conducting a campaign to provide a carton of cigarettes to every patient on Christmas morning. Paul Bolton, one of the campaign participants, wrote the following letter:

> To the Boys in McCloskey General Hospital
> Dear Joe, Jack and Jim:
> Merry Christmas greetings in the form of 3,768 cartons of cigarettes and 5,000 match folders left Austin Tuesday afternoon by bonded express truck. We want you to know that truck is loaded also with good wishes, kind thoughts, a great interest in each of you and our gratitude to you. When we started out asking for a Christmas present of a carton of cigarettes for each of you soldiers in McCloskey, we really expected to get a thousand or so; but more than 3,000 citizens of Austin demanded to be included and letters poured in from all the surrounding territory; so your gift really came from more than 3,000 Central Texas people, each of whom personally remembered you. The last hectic three days of getting the presents ready became a community affair. Several hundred man- and woman-hours were spent Saturday, Sunday and Monday by the wrappers--34 pretty high school girls, who wrapped 2,150 cartons in 43 cases Saturday; the Texas wing of women fliers and the Christian

Endeavor society of the Christian church who took care of 27 more cases. Then five soldiers from Camp Swift, two Texas university naval cadets, and two high school football stars repacked the cases after the wrappers had the cartons fixed up Christmasy. Eight women finished the wrapping job Monday on five cases. We are telling you this so you will see the cross-section of Texas spirit that contributed to this gift--no doubt the largest gift ever sent anywhere from Austin. And the Brown Express company is your immediate Santa Claus, donating the truck, gasoline and men to the delivery job. Nearly every carton has a name on it, one of the people who had a hand in trying to make your Christmas a happier one. If you want to write to the friend who sent your carton and there's no address with the name (putting on the addresses became a clerical mountain we couldn't take), just mail your letter to Paul Bolton, Capitol Station, Austin, and he says he will see that your letters are delivered even though he has to put an ad in the papers. We hope every person connected with the hospital, from Gen. Bethea to the cook's helper, enjoys his smokes. In six days' time, the money poured in so that we couldn't stop at the 3,000 carton goal which was first set; so your medical detachment staff and Red Cross workers are included on our list. Good luck, boys. And remember the spirit behind our gift--expressed over and over, by old and young, rich and poor: "We can't do enough for those boys."
Affectionately yours,
The Citizens of Austin and Central Texas[244]

The following year, the hospital received 208 cedar trees and decorations were sent by people from all over the country. Eighteen-thousand gifts poured in, enough for six gifts per patient. Four thousand pounds of turkey, sixty gallons of oysters, and 1,000 pounds of fruitcake were just a few of the items on the Christmas menu. In 1945, the Belton Chamber of Commerce contributed 105 native cedar trees to McCloskey for use in the wards and auditoriums. A nationwide fundraising effort called Give to a Yank Who Gave, initiated by comedian Eddie Cantor in 1943, also provided Christmas gifts for hospitalized veterans.

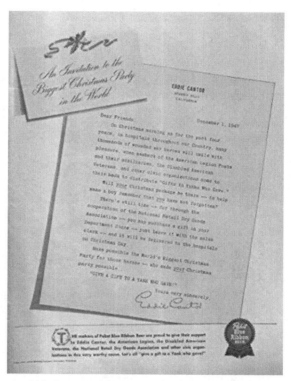

Advertisement featuring Eddie Cantor and Give to A Yank Who Gave. SOURCE: *Life Magazine*, 1947.

The American Legion posts and their auxiliaries, the Disabled American Veterans, and various civic groups partnered at the state level to provide for the war heroes in hospitals in their cities. The Belton American Legion Post No. 55 and its local Auxiliary unit sponsored its own "Gifts for Yanks That Gave" collection in December 1945. Although the war had ended by this time, the post commander, Gilbert Hyer, reminded folks that "many of our sons and daughters will be in hospitals for a long time and it is up to us to make life worthwhile for them during the long hospitalization." W. W. Wendland of Temple, state chairman of the drive, announced that gifts collected in Belton would be sent to Camp Hood while gifts from larger cities would be sent to McCloskey. The American Women's Voluntary Services chapter in Austin made it their goal to remember the patients throughout the year by sending 200 presents each month to McCloskey. Gifts were divided into categories and designated as birthday gifts, game prizes, items to help with rehabilitation, and special gifts for W.A.C.S. They included items such as cigarettes, pipes, leather picture frames, books, shaving lotion, stationery, handkerchiefs, billfolds, fountain pens, and pot plants. The Moslah Shrine Temple of Fort Worth issued an appeal for lawn furniture for the hospital. The A.B.W.A. donated 57 pounds of costume jewelry for use in psychopathic and occupational therapy. The Capitol Lodge of the I.O.O.F. delivered canes and crutches to the hospital contributed by the people of Austin. Miss Emma Wendlandt, chairman of the Red Cross committee in Austin, supervised the collection of over 1,500 coat hangers for the boys at McCloskey. The Texas Federation of Labor collected $2,215 to purchase a new bowling alley and three automatic pinsetters.

McCloskey was the recipient of some unusual gifts as well. Captain Fred. E. Strouse, Quartermaster Sales officer at McCloskey, revealed that a championship steer had been purchased from the Wichita Packing Company in Dallas with the understanding that the meat would be consumed by the patients at the hospital. The steer was raised by Bronnie McNabb and shown at the annual 4-H and F.F.A. Club auction of the Corsicana Livestock and Agricultural Show in September 1944. The grand champion baby beef weighed 1,070 pounds and was purchased by S. N. Georgas of Corsicana who donated the animal to the Navarro County Red Cross. The patients were treated to a rare commodity of high-quality beef, superior to the AA class beef specified by the War Department. In 1945, veterans at the hospital were the beneficiaries of the bidding for the prize steer and other livestock from the Houston Fat Stock Show, totaling more than $8,200.

Another item in the unusual gifts department was a greenhouse paid for by Texas Rotarians. A letter was sent to Rotary Club presidents throughout the state suggesting the building of a structure that would provide shrubs and flowers to beautify the wards and walkways at the hospital. One hundred and fifteen clubs answered the call and sent checks totaling $10,000. General Bethea commissioned Texas A&M College engineers to draw the plans. An Army post engineer supervised construction using prisoner of war labor to pour concrete, work steel, and set glass. The results were a 120-foot long structure with three interior sections of variable temperatures and a sizable room for potting plants. The greenhouse served as a form of occupational therapy to help rehabilitate the veterans. In short order, they were growing everything from asters to zinnias. General Bethea said, "Nothing is more important than giving sick patients beautiful surroundings."[245]

Books and magazines were popular gifts to help patients pass the time. Many area newspapers ran ads soliciting novels and magazines for the McCloskey patients, and occasionally the McCloskey library issued appeals for reading material. Favorite genres included movies, sports, westerns, detective and mystery, and comic books. The patients also enjoyed magazines such as *Life*, *Look*, and the *Saturday Evening Post*. J. M. Dyer Co. of Corsicana featured a McCloskey Hospital Book Depot inside its store to collect donations. Jim McGoldrick of Cameron, in response to a plea in the *Cameron Herald*, collected magazines and took a carload to McCloskey. McGoldrick had the distinction of having delivered more magazines to the hospital than any man in Central Texas. As a member of the American Legion and V.F.W., he volunteered countless hours meeting the needs of the wounded at McCloskey.

Early in 1946, at a meeting of the Central Texas Camp and Hospital Council, Mrs. W. B. Oswald gave details of a new device called a micro-film projector that projected the page of a

145

book onto the ceiling, thus allowing patients to read while lying flat in bed. The Council purchased eight devices from monies donated by Company B of the Texas Rangers in Dallas. Microfilmed books ranged in cost from $1.25 to $1.50 and plans were made to fill the library and promote books of this type. The University of Texas Clipping Bureau created scrapbooks filled with cartoons, jokes, and crossword puzzles for the amusement of the patients.

During the war, the Professional Golfers' Association Rehabilitation Committee expressed its intent to build a series of golf courses for wounded military veterans as well as teach them how to play golf. Major General Norman T. Kirk, the Army's Surgeon General, commended the group for its service to the convalescent patients by providing opportunities for recreation and reconditioning they might not otherwise have. At the state level, *Houston Press* sports editor Ralph Anderson spearheaded efforts to bring outdoor activities to amputees. He had previously constructed a rod and reel for the use of men who had prosthetic arms.[246] Anderson and a group of Houston sportswriters and sportsmen formed the Houston War Sports Activity Committee and approached General Bethea at McCloskey about building a golf course. The General replied, "Build them a golf course." Money was raised quickly through churches, labor unions, liquor salesmen, and fraternal lodges. Each hole was sold for $500.00, and within three days, $7,000.00 had been collected. A nightclub held a special event, charging a set of golf clubs as the price of admission. Seventy sets of clubs were secured. John Bredemus was the commissioned architect for the project, and Major Burns, an engineering officer at McCloskey, oversaw the actual construction, using German P.O.W.s as laborers. Within a short time, a nine-hole course measuring 2,200 yards was designed, and it was purposely constructed to accommodate wheelchair patients. Anderson was so moved by the sight of the amputees playing that he set out to fashion a device to allow a patient to swing a golf club using his prosthesis in concert with his arm. Sergeant Norman Broemel of Pennington, New Jersey, who lost his left arm in Germany, worked with Anderson who developed a leather sleeve with a leather flap that fit around the club's grip. The flap was held in place by the working hand while the hook was inserted into a thong attached to the leather sleeve. On his first attempt, Broemel hit a 5-iron onto the green from 140 yards. One day after winning the Dallas Open in September 1945, Slammin' Sam Snead and Vic Ghezzi demonstrated some of their best golf shots at the dedication of the golf course. The *Abilene Reporter-News* story featured two patients who outshone the pros. After each had missed six straight 15-foot putts, Sergeant Thomas Peterson of Malvern, Pennsylvania, a leg amputee, joined Sergeant Broemel in stepping up to hole putts![247] In 1946, the first annual Veterans Amateur State Golf Championship Tournament was held at the golf course on August 24-25th.[248] Co-sponsored by the hospital's Special Services Office and the Temple Junior Chamber of Commerce, the event was intended to bring the best amateur golfers in the state to play for the veterans and to provide Texas veterans with their own annual sports event. The tourney was open to any amateur golfer who was also a World War I or II veteran. The Jaycees underwrote $225 worth of Victory Bonds for prizes. The Temple Coca-Cola Bottling Company donated a trophy, subsequently called the James A. McCloskey Trophy, on which the winner's name would be inscribed. If a contestant won three years in a row, he would get possession of the trophy; otherwise, it would remain at the hospital. Following the tournament, a free dance for all contestants was held at the McCloskey Employees' Club. For 34 years, the golf course hosted the tournament with golf legends like Byron Nelson, Orville Moody, and Sam Snead in attendance.

In 1943, schoolchildren of Tarrant County, Texas, contributed to the war effort by conducting a nickel and dime campaign to raise funds to purchase land for a lake adjacent to the hospital grounds. Fifty-two acres were purchased for the construction of a park and lake, named Tarrant in honor of the home county of the donors. The project was about one-third completed in 1945 when construction was ordered to cease.

The project ran into trouble when a high-pressure gas line was detected. The park was completed in the 1950s with the help of a Belton Reservoir contractor who donated equipment and manpower to move the gas line. A picnic area with concrete tables and sheltered kitchen areas already existed, built by prisoners of war. Tarrant Lake covered about 11 surface acres, and it was regularly stocked with fish. Both the lake and the park exist today.

General Bethea did his part in soliciting help for hospital improvement on those occasions that he was invited to speaking engagements at various local civic groups. As he often said, "The government does not grant money for beautification."[249] He asked the city of Temple to build waste disposal facilities as well as a sidewalk the length of the hospital so that patients would not have to walk in the street. To beautify the grounds, he asked specifically for pecan and redbud trees as well as red climbing roses for the fence that surrounded the campus. Word spread quickly, and a variety of groups answered the call. The World War II Mothers of Austin made hospital beautification the group's major project and donated 5,000 shrubs and trees and later funded furnishings for the recreational rooms. In a strange turn of events, former governor, James E. Ferguson, requested that upon his death flowers be omitted from the funeral and that living flowers, shrubs, or funds be sent to McCloskey. [250] Ferguson, a native of Bell County, died on September 21, 1944. On his last visit to Temple, he visited the hospital and found it lacking in plantings and expressed a desire to assist in beautifying the grounds. Two Texas university faculty members, F. W. Hensel of Texas A&M and E. J. Urbanovsky of Texas Tech, were appointed to oversee the project and toured the hospital to implement plans with General Bethea. World War II Mothers, the Austin A&M Mothers, the Council of Jewish Women of Austin, the Hyde Park Reading Club of Austin, and various garden clubs got involved. One Austin high school voted to donate $100.00 to purchasing "living shrubs and plants to be set out on the grounds of the hospital at Temple where many Texans are recuperating from

148

battle wounds."[251] In 1945, Mrs. F. A. Huwieler, first vice president of the Texas Garden Clubs, Inc., Mrs. E. W. Frost of Fayetteville, Arkansas, national president of the Garden Clubs, and Mrs. J. H. Berry of Goldthwaite, chairman of War Services for the Texas group, met with General Bethea to discuss their plans for beautification. By 1946, it was estimated that the existing landscaping on the hospital grounds was valued at $160,000. Even as late as 1955, garden clubs were still supplying trees and plants to the McCloskey Veterans Hospital. Women of the Fifth District Division of the Texas Garden Clubs sent 200 young sycamore trees dug from riverbanks in Austin.

The Bell County chapter of the Red Cross played an active role in supporting the patients and staff at McCloskey. Mrs. Margaret Markes, executive secretary of the Red Cross of Bell County, reported to the Belton-Temple A.A.U.W. of the local chapter's accomplishments. From the U.S. entry into the war until September 1, 1942, 756 persons in Bell County had completed first aid courses, 250 had studied nutrition, and 250 had taken home nursing courses.[252] The Production Corps made surgical dressings, glove cases, doctors' and nurses' caps, operating gowns, sheets, and radiator covers for both Camp Hood and McCloskey. A room was set aside in the basement of the courthouse in Belton as a work area for making surgical dressings.   By 1943, Belton ladies were chastised in the newspaper by an anonymous Red Cross worker for falling behind in making surgical dressings:

> If, with constant reminders of what the boys are doing in giving up security, pleasant home surroundings, good jobs and all they may have accomplished in life, the women have grown callous to these reminders, then it should be a matter of community pride, in not letting these much smaller towns and communities so far outstrip Belton in this work.[253]

In 1942, the Red Cross organized a Gray Ladies Hospital and Recreation Corps volunteer group at McCloskey to help ease the loneliness and boredom of being hospitalized. Mary Lela Engvall was one of the organizers of the group.[254] Mrs. Maxwell Murphy directed the volunteers. Services rendered by the Gray Ladies included library work, teaching handicrafts, flower service, shopping, decorating wards for holidays, supplying hostesses for special occasions, and motor transportation. Gray Ladies also read, played games, wrote letters, and tutored patients at McCloskey as well as served as guides for visitors. On Sundays, the Red Cross Motor Corps treated about 30 patients to automobile rides in the countryside and to visit homes and ranches in the area. Mrs. Maynard Robinson, one of Temple's more than 50 Gray Ladies described their work, "We do anything and everything we can." Women who served as volunteers were required to take a course offered by the Red Cross. The course offered in Bell County consisted of 20 lectures and was open to women ages 25 to 56 who were American citizens and members of the Red Cross. In October 1944 the Bell County Red Cross offered its seventh class for Gray Lady training. It included both morning and evening classes for those teachers, employees, and others who worked during the day and a special four-hour class for Junior Gray Ladies, ages 21 to 25. The course of study encompassed ward administration, medical and surgical emergencies, physiotherapy, nursing services, venereal diseases, recreation, and other subjects. Mrs. Murphy made frequent appeals for more members to replace losses in the group which often occurred during hot weather, vacations, and canning season. In July 1945, she stated that the hospital was at its peak load of patients, and 73 Gray Ladies were doing the work formerly done by more than 200.[255] At the end of the year, General Bethea reported that an average of 160 Gray Ladies were available to volunteer every month.[256]

Even after the war ended, the Red Cross continued to have many calls for its services because of needs at McCloskey and Camp Hood. Mrs. Roy (Lida) Langston, committee, chairman of the Motor Corps, reported at the meeting in December 1946 that eight active members had traveled 3,276 miles to assist the canteen corps in providing services such as taking patients Christmas shopping. In another instance, the family of a dying soldier at Camp Hood was rushed from Temple to the post by Red Cross transportation. Other committees gave details on production of surgical dressings for McCloskey as well as disposition of 3,315 army cases, 276 navy cases, and 1,260 ex-servicemen cases during the year. Gray Ladies announced that they were providing ward duty three days each week as well as hosting a coffee hour for patients on Friday nights.[257]

Chapter 9: Seeing Stars

During World War II, at the behest of President Roosevelt, the United Service Organizations (U.S.O.) Camp Shows program assembled units of professional performers and entertainers to cheer the troops serving overseas. U.S.O. Camp Shows, Inc., established a hospital circuit in the states as well. Bob Hope was perhaps the most well-known entertainer whose variety shows traveled to overseas war zones as well as to military camps and hospital wards in the states. Other Hollywood celebrities toured the country, performing and promoting the sale of war bonds, raising money for servicemen's relief funds, and boosting morale of the injured and infirm.

Throughout the war, McCloskey General Hospital was featured in hundreds of news stories and photographs. The Public Relations Office and Signal Corps were a beehive of activity, spreading the word about McCloskey by distributing photographs and press releases to magazines, newspapers, and networks. The Signal Corps provided 372 photographs in 1944 alone, many of which were picked up by the Associated Press. People all over the country read human interest stories about McCloskey General Hospital in their local newspapers. The P.R. office also published informational booklets, sent notices of awards and promotions to patients' hometown newspapers, and produced radio programs and spot announcements. Commander Bethea's motto of *"Happiness, Kindness and Efficiency"* served as the title of a 24-page photo collage booklet given to incoming patients to introduce them to all the units at the hospital.

McCloskey received its share of famous and not-so-famous entertainers and visitors. All visiting celebrities were escorted through the hospital, interviewed, and photographed. Stories and pictures were sent out on each celebrity. Numerous politicians and Hollywood stars made calls on the veterans. Representative Will Rogers, Jr. was present when 250 wounded from the Southwest Pacific theater of war reached their hospital destination in Temple. Gale Sondergaard, an actress who was originally cast as the wicked witch in *The Wizard of Oz* movie took time to eat lunch with soldiers in the mess hall at McCloskey in April 1944. Governor Coke Stevenson visited McCloskey in 1943 in conjunction with the dedication of a U.S.O. center in Temple and found the patients happily showing off their new arms and legs. Luis L. Duplan, consul of Mexico, commented on the splendid morale of the patients during his visit in February 1944. General Fred L. Walker, who led the Texas 36th Division to victories in Africa and Italy, toured the state visiting his wounded men in various Army hospitals and was met with "affectionate regard and cordiality."[258] Even Congressman Lyndon Johnson referenced McCloskey patients when citizens on the home front complained to him about hardships. "You'll find some without arms to reach for a cup of coffee, some without hands to stir a spoonful of sugar... some without hearing, but you'll also find they are cheerful, unbeaten men!"[259]

Helen Keller and her traveling companion, Polly Thompson, spent time with amputees at McCloskey in 1944 and posed for a photograph. Keller had a special empathy for those blinded in the war, and after visiting as many as 90 hospitals, she became an avid supporter of legislation for funding of rehabilitation and vocational programs for blind and maimed servicemen. She told a friend,

> As Polly and I journeyed through Arkansas, Oklahoma, Texas, New Mexico, Colorado, Utah, California, Oregon and Washington we were kept high-strung by the miracles of rehabilitation we saw. Hospitals which would once have been places of heartbreak are today bright with a dynamic faith and the purpose it inspires. Wounded soldiers who a few years ago were thought doomed are regaining health, interest in

living and self-confidence to reshape their future.
260

Following her visit, General Bethea wrote a letter to Miss Keller thanking her, saying "You carried away the hearts of us all" and for bringing joy to the hospital patients. He quoted one patient as saying, "I thought I was disabled and handicapped until I met Helen Keller. Now I know my handicaps can be overcome."[261]

Like many other singers and entertainers, Gene Autry, joined the military and his Melody Ranch Radio Show became the Sergeant Gene Autry Radio Show as he continued his music and comedy routines with special patriotic music and sketches reflecting military life. Autry also visited numerous army hospitals where he entertained patients. He was well-received at McCloskey, and Lieutenant Ralph S. McGill and Corporal Woodrow Brown were photographed talking with him. Another serviceman, Bobby Byrne, served in the Air Force and while stationed at the Eagle Pass Army Airfield in Texas, led the top-rated dance band, the Skyliners, of the Eighth Service Command. Lieutenant Byrne was called "The Young Man with a Horn." The band skyrocketed to success in 1941 and made several appearances at McCloskey during the war.[262]

From all around the state, various groups made sure the patients were entertained and appreciated throughout the year. Members of the Westwood Country Club in Houston led by *Houston Press* sportswriter, Andy Anderson, arranged for weekend entertainment for five or six veterans at a time. An expense fund of several thousand dollars was dedicated to furnishing all the comforts of home and a whirl of entertainment for the guests. The veterans were housed in a luxurious dormitory in the clubhouse where all their needs were provided for including hometown newspapers delivered every morning. Every imaginable fun-filled activity was offered such as fishing in a well-stocked lake, golfing, hunting, football games, dancing, movies, banquets, and even entertainment in private homes. Westwood's mission was to help the veterans forget their handicaps and to ease the transition to civilian life. A group of five McCloskey vets were entertained on Thanksgiving weekend in 1944 and were captured in a newspaper photograph.

The Rotarians of Texas City held an annual Disabled Veterans Day, and its first group of honorees came from McCloskey. In the January 1946 *Rotarian* magazine, an article entitled *"48 Hours in Paradise"* by Lieutenant Thomas F. Sliger wrote of how much the trip meant to him and his hospital buddies. The group consisted of eight "bilaterals" (men with both legs gone), five of them in wheelchairs and three walking on artificial limbs. After being introduced to their "dates," the men were driven with police escort to a barbeque and swimming party. According to Sliger, there was food and plenty of it including two-inch-thick Texas steaks. The next day, they boarded a U.S. Engineers tugboat for a fishing trip in Galveston Bay. Upon docking, there was a beach party and a shrimp dinner. A moonlight cruise took them back to Texas City. On Sunday, a fishing trip was followed by a grand farewell dinner. Sliger summed up by saying, "No one could have packed more into 48 hours than did those Texas City Rotarians. None of us had a moment even to think that we were disabled. None of us will ever forget that trip."[263] A similar trip was sponsored by the Houston Metal Trades Council and four major oil companies for 10 Purple Heart recipients from McCloskey. The servicemen's cruise in four palatial yachts provided by local physicians was the highlight of a fun-filled weekend that also included a fish fry, dance, and horse show.[264] Wardell H. Creamer, Temple bus line executive, invited four amputees on a hunting trip where they proved that their physical handicaps had not affected their ability to shoot. Roy Differding of Walker, Iowa; Clarence Barthelemy of Bushnell, Florida; Andrew Weslowski of Milwaukee Wisconsin; and Abe Beal of Springfield, Missouri bagged five bucks and a wild turkey.[265]

Closer to home, the Cole Brothers Circus came to Temple in October 1944. A complete ring with clowns, trapezists, tightrope performers, elephants, and horses set up camp on the hospital grounds east of the admission building. Special acts from the circus also toured the wards to entertain the patients. School groups and choirs commonly traveled through Texas visiting army hospitals and presenting vocal music. The following month, the Musical Charm Program, a 50-member student entertainment group from Texas State College of Women in Denton, made its debut at McCloskey. T.S.C.W., known for its variety shows, regularly entertained servicemen at hospitals around the state. In a previous visit to McCloskey the girls' morale-building efforts in the hospital wards were so welcomed that General Bethea asked for a return engagement. One of the most popular shows was presented by Stage Door Canteen. The Stage Door Canteen originated in the Broadway theater district with the aim of providing dancing, entertainment, food, and nonalcoholic drinks for servicemen from all branches of the armed forces. By 1945 all the canteens closed, and attention shifted to providing entertainment and recreation in hospital settings. The Temple show, described as the "finest entertainment ever given at McCloskey," featured Adele Lambert who frequently appeared at the New York Stage Door Canteen. Other stars on the program included Joanne Farrar (dancer), Betty Andress (accordionist), Frances Koonsen (singer), and Dave Jeffry of Camp Swift who was accompanied by a chorus of eight girls with music provided by the McCloskey hospital orchestra. Forty hostesses from Smithville, Taylor, and Austin furnished smiles and conversation. The evening ended with the audience singing, "I Left My Heart at the McCloskey Canteen."

One group of entertainers was not allowed to perform at McCloskey. A group of teenage canteen performers from Mexia, Texas, asked to stage a black-face minstrel show at the hospital. Captain Faraon Moss, public relations officer, stated that hospital officials considered the show "inappropriate for a mixed audience of wounded white and Negro troops." A similar performance two years earlier brought protests. Officials at McCloskey denied reports that the cancellation was due to a War Department ban on black-face minstrel entertainment for wounded servicemen. The War Department backed McCloskey declaring "there has been absolutely no such order."[266] The show was held in Temple at the City Auditorium with free admission for servicemen. Camp Hood and McCloskey General Hospital played a role in what would later be called a symbol of the civil rights movement. Jackie Robinson, the all-star athlete, was drafted by the army in April 1942 and was sent to Fort Riley, Kansas. Soon thereafter, he was reassigned to the 761st "Black Panther" Tank Battalion at Camp Hood. Lieutenant Robinson, who had a bad ankle, had a status of "limited duty" and was sent to McCloskey hospital for evaluation and treatment to determine his fitness to go overseas. On July 6, 1944, he boarded a city bus to go to Temple and then on to Camp Hood where he spent time at the Officer's Club. On his return trip to McCloskey, the lieutenant ran into trouble with Milton Reneger, the driver for the Southwestern Bus Company, who told Robinson to move to the rear of the bus. A chaotic string of events followed with Robinson being arrested and returned to McCloskey under guard. He remained confined to quarters until his court martial on August 2, 1944 when he was acquitted of all charges.[267]

The Red Cross played a big role in providing entertainment for patients. The Red Cross buildings at McCloskey contained two auditoriums with seating capacities of 500 and 750 where first-run movies were shown, and musical programs were held including a symphony concert. Monthly birthday parties with refreshments quickly became a tradition with 200-300 patients in attendance, but the activities that drew the most interest were quiz games and bingo.

The local U.S.O. clubs provided entertainment for the McCloskey vets as well. Frequent articles appeared in local newspapers of the time reporting on their activities. In conjunction with the Chamber of Commerce, the Belton U.S.O. treated 47 ambulatory and wheelchair patients to the Fourth of July rodeo in 1945 followed by a fried chicken dinner. Patients especially enjoyed outings and weekend trips. On November 11, 1944, a group of McCloskey vets was gifted with a trip to the Texas Technical vs. Texas Christian University football game and

Private First Class Denver Morris (Burk, TX.); Sergeant Herbert Cauley (Kingsville, TX.); and Private First Class John A. Hecht (New York City, NY.) were pictured in the stands enjoying the game. Forty McCloskey patients attended the Cotton Bowl football game in Dallas in January 1946. Their lodging was provided at the Melrose Hotel where they were guests at a banquet in their honor. C. R. McDilda, director of the Belton U.S.O., entertained the group with a magic show. The Red Cross Motor Corps girls transported veterans to various activities around the state, including the Southwestern Exhibition and Fat Stock Show in Fort Worth. First Sergeant Don Simpson, a patient at McCloskey, had the opportunity to meet Bud Linderman, a bronc rider in the show and a World War II veteran.

Holidays were special times and might include movies, fall bonfires, wiener roasts, and outdoor games. There was always a big Christmas party each year with gifts being donated by local merchants. To meet increasing needs of convalescents at the hospital, the Belton U.S.O. announced an expansion in May 1945 to include a retaining wall and terraced playground equipped with concrete picnic tables, badminton court, and a future boat landing on the city lake. Soon after, the Variety Club of Dallas offered use of its grounds and facilities west of Belton for recreation and weekend activities for the patients. The U.S.O. club even served as a wedding chapel for one McCloskey patient who was married at the Belton U.S.O. in 1945 with Adjutant McDilda officiating. Private First Class John J. Oroszy of Conneaut, Ohio, and Miss Frances Leone Lerwill of Portland, Oregon, were married before an improvised altar of red roses and ferns. [268] About 100 guests were in attendance, 30 of them fellow patients of the bridegroom. The bride was given in marriage by her mother and carried a white satin Bible with pink and white carnations. The bookmark was a cord from the bridegroom's parachute. Sergeant Tommy Cunningham of Camp Hood sang "Always in My Heart" and Miss Betty Ann McDilda sang "Because." Miss Rosetta Howard was maid of honor with Patricia Ann Faulkner as flower girl and Robert Dillard as ring bearer. A wedding reception was held at the

Variety Club with Dallas officials of the Variety Club Foundation present for the festivities. The following Thanksgiving, the U.S.O. hosted activities at the Variety Camp where 30 men from McCloskey spent the holiday weekend horseback riding, hunting, and fishing, capped by a traditional turkey dinner.

Many other activities were planned to entertain the patients and keep their minds occupied. The first annual bathing beauty contest to select "Miss McCloskey" was held at the opening of the new swimming pool in 1944. The contest was open to all women personnel employed on the post and wives of the enlisted men of the 1884th Service Command. Prominent local citizens served as judges, and Mary Louise Carper won the title. A picnic supper and pool party were held in conjunction with the contest. Joy Hudspeth was named "Miss McCloskey" the following year.

In October 1944, the publisher E.P. Dutton announced the G.I. Joe Literary Award for the best manuscript by a service man or woman, whether officer or enlisted, who had been wounded in action in the war. Awards were planned for 1945, 1946, and 1947, and a prize of $5,000 given. An advisory council was appointed to select the best manuscript which should be not less than 50,000 words in length and could include fiction, non-fiction, short stories, or poetry. Members of the council were Captain Robert D. Workman, Colonel Franklin S. Forsberg, Sergeant Marion Hargrove, John Hersey, and Lieutenant John Mason Brown. The judges who made the final decision were George Moreby Acklom, Fred T. Marsh, and J. Donald Adams. The library at McCloskey provided pamphlets and posters with details of the contest and placed books on writing on display for use by the patients. The patients were also eligible to enter the Thomas Jefferson Southern Award contest and the Lewis and Clark Northwest contest, each with a prize of $2,500 McCloskey held its own contest earlier in the year with cash awards going to five patients at the hospital for their poetry: Private Homer Labee (Caldwell, ID.); Sergeant Walter M. Graham (San Antonio, TX.); Private First Class Antony Nicosia (Allentown, PA.); T. L. Hyde (Abilene, TX.); and Sergeant T. C. English of Ohio. The winning poems were read over the Blue Network on Ted Malone's *Between the Bookends* program.

McCloskey found a way to give back to the community when the 79th Army Ground Forces band was assigned to the hospital. The band arrived at Temple on November 27, 1944, from Fort Crockett and was composed of 28 enlisted men. It was organized in 1942 as an integral part of the 20th Coast Artillery Regiment under the direction of Chief Warrant Officer Marion E. Durbin and designated and attached to the harbor defenses of Galveston. Called the 442nd Army Service Forces Band, its specialty was martial and dance music. The band spent two and a half years in field training for overseas services. At home, most of the band's engagements included recreational activities such as dances, parades, guard mounts, W.A.C. recruiting, and bond shows as well as many broadcasts over radio station KLUF Galveston. Once in Temple, the band made its first appearance in a war bond parade in December 1944 and later in the Belton Fourth of July Parade in 1945. The Belton Chamber of Commerce contributed $50 to the band fund in appreciation for its participation.

McCloskey was often the site of a variety of radio broadcasts and an intercommunication system allowed patients on the wards to listen in. The McCloskey band was featured in a KTEM radio program called "Meet the Men of McCloskey," beamed from the hospital, which presented patient talent and interviews with members of the hospital staff and battle casualties recently returned from combat zones. The local programming was conceived by Burton Bishop, manager of KTEM, and organized by hospital officials. A program created by Norman J. Dickens of WBAP in Fort Worth called "McCloskey Speaks" was another means toward helping the men return to normal civilian life. Mayor Guy Draper of Temple heartily endorsed the program, stating, "it gives the public a clear picture of what the returned veteran is facing when he returns to civilian status. I believe that the program is equal to any I have ever heard and superior to most because the personnel used are recently returned veterans from various battlefronts and their interviews and stories are up to date."[269] The program format consisted of patient interviews during which they spoke candidly about their problems, their hopes and dreams for the future, and the work they would like to do upon returning to civilian life. Many had to face the harsh reality that returning to their former occupations would be impossible and were seeking sincere advice regarding the reshaping of their future. The response from the public was overwhelming with hundreds of letters received offering suggestions, help, and even jobs. Staff Sergeant Hal Motheral of San Marcos appeared on one broadcast where he stated he had been employed by an oil well supply company in south Texas. He received a job offer and a card from an Oklahoman suggesting he run for Congress. Private William H. Edwards of Hayti expressed a desire to buy a small farm in Texas.[270] Private J. C. Chambless of Oklahoma City aspired to be a professional baseball player before the war. The 19-year-old paratrooper lost his right foot and the toes on his left foot when a German SS officer took his jump boots and left him without shoes. Staff Sergeant George Hart from Dallas hoped to own a garage and service station on a popular highway heading to New Mexico. In a speech to the Texas Associated Press Managing Editors Association in Dallas in 1945, Captain Faraon J. Moss told the attendees that of the 20,000 men discharged from McCloskey, each one had been offered a *bona fide* job. Passage of the Serviceman's Readjustment Act of 1944 (G.I. Bill of Rights) further aided veterans in getting jobs, pursuing education, and helping them readjust to civilian life.

In 1945, two national radio broadcasts over CBS and NBC emanated directly from the hospital, one of which was the popular "Coca-Cola Parade of Spotlight Bands" program. While on tour, Frankie Masters and his orchestra broadcast from McCloskey. Masters and his band held the record for the most (57) appearances on the show. From McCloskey he went on to entertain the men stationed at Love Field. Occasionally veterans represented McCloskey on "Army Showtime," a weekly program broadcast over the Texas Quality Network. Arnold F. Murdock, recipient of the Purple Heart for wounds received at Salerno in

161

the 36th Division, received Showtime's Banner of Fame in October 1944. Other patients who were mentioned included Leland C. Grohman of San Antonio who lost his left arm; Ewing Mays of Heber Springs, Arkansas, a member of the Rangers who lost both legs; and Richard Reno of Pecan Gap, Robert Thad Knittel, Jr. of Burton, and James C. Carpenter, all wounded in the Italian campaign.

It was not unusual for the wounded war heroes to take part in bond campaigns around the state. In January 1944, men from the Texas 36th Division made appearances in Austin at various civic clubs and a bond rally arranged by the Austin Junior Chamber of Commerce. Men who helped launch the bond campaign were Private First Class Wallace Watson (Winters, TX.), Private First Class Tom Starr (Ballinger, TX.), Private First Class George G. Nelson (Crisfield, MD.), 1st Lieutenant Homer E. Cluck (Amarillo, TX.), Master Sergeant Clinton R. Eaton (Amarillo, TX.), and Lieutenant Colonel Joseph E. McShane (San Antonio, TX.). Dignitaries in attendance were Governor Coke Stevenson, Mayor Tom Miller, and Harfield K. Weedin, master of ceremonies. Lunch music was provided by Technical Sergeant Jack Ream's Bergstrom Army Airfield Orchestra. The meeting was designed to arouse enthusiasm among the citizens in order to raise $6,965 for the Fourth War Loan Drive.[271] The following month, the first Flying Fortress B-17 landed in Temple to transport veterans to Ardmore, Oklahoma, for a bond drive. Later in the year, the McCloskey vets again urged citizens to buy bonds in the Fifth War Loan Drive. It was reported that by speaking at meetings and bond rallies throughout the Eighth Service Command, the patients were indirectly responsible for $194,776.704 in bond sales. One hundred forty-five patients including 25 officers and 120 enlisted men recounted their personal battle experiences at 511 meetings.[272] The employees of the hospital also raised $123,895.13 in the bond drive. As part of the campaign for the Fifth War Loan Drive, the hospital PR Office prepared pictures and story materials for a special display at Neiman-Marcus in Dallas featuring thirty-nine store windows depicting actual battle scenes. For the sixth bond drive, the

162

hospital exceeded its former quota by purchasing $150,844.74 in bonds.[273] In his final annual report, General Bethea wrote that wounded soldiers, including 141 officers and 326 enlisted men, appeared at 261 patriotic rallies in behalf of the war effort in 1945. They were directly or indirectly responsible for the sale of $448,212,212.00 worth of war bonds during the previous three years.[274]

Some organizations held auctions or shows to raise money for bonds. A war bond wrestling show held in Dallas in June 1944 featured celebrities including Jack Dempsey and Gene Autry. Bill Longson, world heavyweight wrestling champ, defeated Jack Kennedy in the main event of the show. Mrs. Eleanor Gehrig, wife of the famous baseball player, Lou Gehrig, contributed her husband's 1936 American League's Most Valuable Player trophy through her brother, Private First Class Frank Twitchell of the Fifth Ferrying Group stationed in Dallas. The winning bidder was the Southland Life Insurance Company of Dallas, paying $1 million dollars in bond purchases. Southland, in turn, presented the trophy to the patients at McCloskey General Hospital. Mrs. Gehrig, who donated various pieces of her husband's memorabilia for war bond sales during the war, expressed surprise at the sum generated, and in a telegram said, "This may save a life." [275] The whereabouts of the trophy are unknown.

Stellar medical care coupled with the kindness and caring expressed by people both far and near undoubtedly contributed to the cheery spirit dominant in the hospital. Raymond Brooks, a reporter for *The Austin American-Statesman,* visited 30 wards at McCloskey in August 1944. He wrote,

> [My] first, last and composite impression was of the tremendously buoyant, cheerful and forward-looking spirit of the group of patients, the dynamic health and vigor of the men, apart from specific wounds or maiming injury. There are

soldiers who have lost legs, those who
have lost an arm, or an eye; those
wounded in every way that searing,
exploding steel can tear a human body.
And this certainly is not intended to make
light   of the wound that costs a man a
leg or otherwise maims him for life. The
point is that if a man is to lose his leg, the
spirit at McCloskey is that something else
as important as the leg is the cheery, self-
reliant, calm, forward-looking spirit of the
men.   Those   men   aren't   wanting
sympathy.[276]

Similar sentiments were expressed by a *Denison Press*
newspaperman who visited McCloskey and assured the
mothers, wives, and sweethearts that their lads were being
cared for "better than any soldiers ever were cared for before."

They are getting the best medical and
surgical attention that can be had. And,
best of all, they are loved and lovingly
cared for by the officers, nurses, and men
who staff this great army healing unit.
There is nothing impersonal about the
way McCloskey Hospital takes care of its
boys. Every patient is a personal
responsibility of those who staff the great
institution, and nothing is left undone to
return them to health, happiness, and
usefulness. [277]

He was led on his tour of the hospital by the public relations
officer, Captain Moss, who quipped at the boys and called
almost everyone by name. He spent hours chatting with the
patients about their part in the fighting. He met Corporal Leland
Grohman of San Antonio who praised the U.S.O. for sending

camp shows overseas to entertain the boys. Sergeant Charlie Rummell of Waco who had been a prisoner of war praised the National War Fund and War Prisoners Aid for providing sports equipment, books, and other materials to the Nazi prison camps. He encountered two women, Lieutenant Marjorie Gray of Killeen, and Lieutenant Helen McCullough, nurses who were recuperating at McCloskey from duty at Anzio. Among them all, he found nothing but cheerful courage and was inspired by their bravery and sacrifice.

Chapter 10: Barbed Wire and Black Tar Paper

When the United States entered World War II following the bombing of Pearl Harbor, prison camps in the United Kingdom were overflowing, and the government appealed to the Americans for help. The U.S. agreed, somewhat reluctantly, to use its Liberty Ships to transport Axis prisoners of war to the mainland. Near the end of 1943, Secretary of War, Henry Stimson, revealed that 140,000 prisoners of war were in the United States. Of those, about 100,000 were Germans; the remaining number were Italians. The basics of the Geneva Convention of 1929 stipulated how prisoners of war were to be treated. The guidelines stated that camps had to be comparable to U.S. army camps with food, clothing, medical care, and recreation thoughtfully determined. Some work could also be required of prisoners if it met certain requirements. The U.S. government was careful to adhere to the stipulations and ensure that German P.O.W.s were well-treated, hoping that American prisoners in Germany would receive corresponding treatment. The Army Corps of Engineers began a vigorous building program with recommendations for what constituted an "ideal" camp: 350 acres in size away from populated areas; clearly defined perimeter with guard towers and barbed wire; capacity of 2,000- 4,000 prisoners, divided into four compounds of 500-700 men; and each compound having four barracks, a mess hall, a workshop, a canteen, an infirmary, an administrative building, a recreation hall, an inspection ground, a processing center and a soccer field.[278] The U.S. government further required that camps had to be 170 miles from the coasts, 150 miles from the Canadian or Mexican borders, and away from munitions factories, shipyards and any other war related industries. A total of 155 base camps were built. Smaller branch camps were built predominantly in the South and Midwest to locate prisoners close to areas where labor was needed. By the end of the war, there were a total of 511 camps spread all over the country.

The War Department established the Prisoner of War Employment Reviewing Board to oversee the use of P.O.W. labor. Upon arrival in the United States, prisoners were transported by train to the camps. Originally P.O.W. labor was intended for use on military bases, but as time went on, the government recognized that help was needed in industry and agriculture. The wartime draft of farmers or their sons had depleted the farm labor supply and Secretary of Agriculture Wickard ordered an inventory of men and women who were suitable for such work. In cases where civilian labor was unavailable, farmers could apply for prisoner-of-war labor to the commanders of the internment camps who were authorized to negotiate contracts on behalf of the War Department.

Texas had twice as many prisoner-of-war camps as any other state, housing over 50,000 German prisoners. Three branch camps were built in Texas specifically to provide prisoner labor for general hospitals at McCloskey General Hospital in Temple, Ashburn General Hospital in McKinney, and Harmon General Hospital in Longview. Camp McCloskey was the first to be established, opening in October 1944.[279] It was considered a branch camp of the prisoner-of-war camp at Camp Hood.

Temple's camp was located across the street from the main campus at the current site of Temple College on the west side of South 1st Street. The encampment was sometimes referred to by locals as "Black City" because of its black tar-paper-covered huts. The camp consisted of two barracks buildings, a mess hall, and administrative offices.[280] Each barrack was divided into about 20 rooms with three cots per room. In March 1945, an inspection by State Department official, Vanarsdale Turner, noted that barracks were terribly overcrowded by trying to cram too many prisoners into each room.[281] One local resident described the camp with "rolled up barbed wire all around it with guards in big tall stands with the biggest, ugliest guns you've ever seen." Most of the prisoners were German veterans from the Africa campaign. Italian prisoners were sent elsewhere since they and the Germans did not get along.

Upon their arrival, prisoners of war were put to work. Maintenance work on the buildings and grounds was the primary type of labor performed by P.O.W.s at Camp McCloskey. When the hospital first opened it was lacking paved streets so many German P.O.W.s were enlisted to construct roads on the south side of the hospital. Some prisoners worked inside the hospital, waxing floors and cleaning but contact with patients was forbidden. Other prisoners could serve as orderlies in the prisoner-of-war wing of the hospital.[282]

During the first nine months of 1944, prisoner-of-war patients admitted to the hospital were German and Italian with the German nationality predominating five-to-one. On September 16, 1944, all German patients needing more than two weeks hospitalization were transferred to Glennan General Hospital in Okmulgee, Oklahoma, and thereafter it became the policy to transfer all those who required prolonged hospitalization. Occasionally short-term emergency admissions were allowed from camps in the area. In September and October of 1944, about 200 Russian, Polish, Czechoslovakian, and Yugoslavian battle casualties were admitted. The 1944 annual report indicated that 583 prisoner-of-war patients were admitted and 483 were discharged that year.[283]

The Internal Security Section of the hospital was responsible for all activities related to those prisoners who were admitted to the hospital, and all personnel assigned were carefully selected. Some were able to speak various foreign languages to assist in obtaining medical histories and other information. The P.O.W. patients on the wards were always guarded by a detail of 29 men who rotated through various P.O.W. camps and were sent to the hospital for a thirty-day period. General Bethea said the P.O.W.s received the same care as other patients in the hospital. In 1944, a news report told of a German prisoner of war who was beaten by fellow prisoners at Camp Hearne. He was rescued by guards and transported to McCloskey where he died from his injuries on December 23, 1943.[284]

Each morning, prisoners marched to the hospital grounds where they were divided into work groups and assigned an escort. Temple resident, Douglas Truesdale, served in the military police during the war and often accompanied prisoners when they were transferred to McCloskey or to other concentration camps in Hearne or Mexia. It was customary to transfer prisoners to various camps to prevent them from forming cliques or causing trouble. Truesdale recalled guarding prisoners with a shotgun as they worked on the hospital grounds, building the gymnasium and swimming pool. Prisoners planted approximately 30,000 permanent shrubs and 1,000 trees. *The Austin American-Statesman* reported that many of the prisoners had been farmers in Germany and were well-suited to outdoor landscaping work. On one particular hot day when marching back to their quarters, lightning struck a squad of German prisoners, killing one.

The late Mrs. Mary Farrell, a history professor at Temple Junior College, said in a 1985 interview that prisoners who were enlisted men could work around town. "I never heard of anybody objecting to them working in town," Farrell said. In a 1999 interview with the *Temple Daily Telegram*, Lottie Fowler, who worked at McCloskey during the war, described interacting with German soldiers. "Some of them were cooks and they taught me how to make twisted rolls, all kinds of things. I was 16, going on 17 at the time, and they were very friendly to work with. They never caused any trouble that I can recall."[285] Some locals grumbled at what they perceived was the healthy appearance of the German prisoners in Temple as compared with the malnourished condition of American soldiers in German P.O.W. camps.

An outdoor handball court, the first of its kind in Temple, provided recreation for the prisoners. They were also occasionally treated to musical entertainment. One such occasion was when Mildred "Lanky" Lancaster was invited to the camp to play the accordion for the German prisoners. Mildred was a junior in high school and one of the few females to step foot inside the camp. Her story is well-known:

When I got inside, the POWs were sitting in straight-back chairs facing straight ahead. They had their hands at the sides. They couldn't clap even if they wanted to. I didn't know what to play. I was sort of over to the side and I didn't know what they wanted to hear. They weren't allowed to say anything. So, I started thinking Seaton, Sefcik Hall. I played 'Beer Barrel Polka.' They couldn't say anything, but I looked in their eyes and I could tell that was just the kind of thing they wanted to hear.[286]

Records of the prisoner-of-war camp were classified, and it is not known if there were any escapes from Camp McCloskey. However, stories of escapes from nearby Camp Hood which housed 4,000 prisoners-of-war, appeared in newspapers across the country. In June 1943, the *Santa Cruz Sentinel* told of the escape of five German prisoners from the camp. FBI agents were called in to help local officials search for the escapees. Two were captured in Cedar Park by civilians. Later that year, in September, four prisoners, who were cutting wood between the towns of Mound and Flat, made a getaway from north Camp Hood. A general radio alarm was sent out for the four who were dressed in khaki dyed blue with "PW" seals on the trousers, blouse, and both arms. Only one of the quartet spoke English. Two of the four were treed by bloodhounds and captured eight miles north of Copperas Cove. Another incident was reported in January 1945 when three prisoners escaped from a work detail. The Department of Public Safety broadcast a warning that the three were "considered dangerous." In May 1944, a report issued by Colonel Daniel B. Byrd of the Eighth Service Command assured citizens that all escapees from camps in the five-state service command area had been recaptured. The colonel remarked "They just don't understand the size of this country. They get away but they don't get far."[287]

From 1942-1945, there were approximately 400,000 prisoners of war housed in the 511 camps spread throughout the country.[288] German P.O.W.s performed 90,629,233 man days of labor just on military bases between 1943 and 1945.[289] The prisoners of war were quickly repatriated as soon as the war ended. In January 1945, there were 41,455 in Texas; by January of the following year, there were 23,987, and repatriation was expected to be completed by the end of April 1946.[290] Harvesting and processing of cotton, sugar cane, rice, and pulpwood were the most important tasks completed by the P.O.W.s in Texas. They filled a critical need created by the war, and the labor they performed at McCloskey General Hospital made a significant contribution with the addition of new facilities and beautification of the grounds. Sadly, today there are virtually no remnants of the camps, including the one in Temple, the remains of which are buried under a parking lot.

Chapter 11: War Stories

Although it was in a small central Texas town, McCloskey General Hospital received visitors, patients, and employees from around the world. Its cast of characters was commanded throughout by one man, Colonel (later General) James A. Bethea. In his memoirs, he marveled at the opportunities that came to him as the hospital commander:

> On the more pleasant side of running a big hospital during the war was the opportunity to meet so many fine people. I refer not only to the large number of wonderful people who were devoting full time to healing the battle casualties, but also to the prominent individuals who came from all over the United States (and elsewhere) to entertain and cheer up those who had been crippled by the war. Among the many personalities whom I got to meet and talk with in this way were the man who is now the President of the United States, a Swedish princess, the Governor of Texas, Helen Keller, many well-known actors and actresses from Hollywood, and others too numerous to mention.[291]

Thousands of people traveled the halls and grounds of McCloskey General Hospital during the war years. It saw patients from every battlefield of the war, and its corridors were like the world's crossroads for men and women from Munda and Attu, from Tunisia and Sicily, from Salerno and Cassino, from Bougainville and Kwajalein, and outposts in India, China, and the Caribbean. Walter Humphrey, the editor of the *Temple Daily Telegram,* was often present when convoys arrived at all hours of the day or night to interview the incoming men and file stories for the folks back home. The stories and recollections captured in books and newspaper articles of the time reveal brief glimpses of the individuals who passed through the hospital's doors. Those presented here represent only a selected few of the hundreds of personal interest stories written.

As battle-scarred soldiers arrived at the hospital, many were eager to tell their personal accounts of events. One such group of men, from Texas' own 36th Division, told of the harrowing landing at Salerno, Italy, in September 1943. Sergeant Charles McFarland of Killeen, member of a Belton infantry unit, confirmed that the 36th Division was the first American force to step on Italian soil, and instead of surprising the Germans, they were met by machine-gun fire. McFarland was wounded in the chest. Private Robert Rawlins of Snyder said the Germans were waiting in the hills everywhere. Rawlins received a severe concussion that day but managed to fight on for seven more days before his injuries forced him out of action. Private George Pollock of Groesbeck credited the air force with turning the tide of the invasion. Corporal Thomas Hovenkamp of Fort Worth told of riding in a Higgins boat, landing on the beach, and being wounded in the leg by shrapnel after going two miles inland. Private Alvis Sims of Groesbeck said he thought it was a dream when he was told he was being sent to Temple. "I'm afraid I'll wake up tomorrow and find I'm back in Italy or North Africa."[292] Sims was wounded six miles inland and had to wait eight hours before being picked up.

Several high-ranking officers of the Fifth Army were among 60 men who arrived at McCloskey from Stark General Hospital in April 1944, with fresh accounts of terrible fighting from Salerno to Anzio. Both Colonel James C. Styron of Hobart, Oklahoma, and Lieutenant Colonel Andy Price of Fort Worth told of the Texas 36th Division's fight against odds which decimated its strength. "The beachhead was level and under constant fire. The Germans would see every move and lay it on you."[293] Also in the convoy was Private Edward E. Elliott of Temple who recounted how a shell hit an olive tree over his head and the shell fragments hit him in both feet and legs. One unexpected event for which the medical officers on the train were unprepared occurred when a nurse with the Fifth Army gave birth to a daughter. It caused "quite a bit of consternation" on the train. One good Samaritan lost his leg when carrying a wounded comrade to safety. Private Edward J. Holt, a 36th Division rifleman, was less concerned about the loss of his limb than how to break the news to his wife, Iva Louise. He neglected to mention his disability in his letters, but when she arrived at McCloskey, she exclaimed, "Oh, Sonny, I'm so proud of you. You didn't have to tell me about it. I knew it all the time." [294] Gordon P. Roman of Longview related his experiences as his division followed the 36th Division into Rome in June 1944. Roman reported that Texans moved into hotels in the city while Germans still had control. The following day when Roman arrived, Italian citizens were wild with joy, filled the soldiers' canteens with wine and cold water, and gave them oranges and fruit. The highlight for Roman was swimming in Mussolini's private pool where a nearby statue of the dictator stood with its head decapitated.[295]

In July 1944, the first invasion casualties from Normandy reached McCloskey and included artillery, infantry, paratroopers, and glider infantry. They were flown across the Atlantic on July 4 and then from Mitchell Field, New York, to Temple. Some were too seriously wounded to be interviewed, but Walter Humphrey was able to talk to some men as they waited to be unloaded to ambulances. Lieutenant Ralph S. McGill of Fort Worth told his story. On D-Day, he parachuted into France and broke both ankles when he landed. He and others were held by the Germans at a field hospital until being rescued by the Ninth Division.[296]

Seventeen Texans were among twenty-seven U.S. officers and enlisted men from German prison camps who were exchanged through the International Red Cross and transported to the States on the Swedish exchange liner *Gripsholm* in February 1945. They arrived at McCloskey in March with Captain M. L. Monroe of Beaumont heading the group. Monroe, a battalion surgeon with the 36th Division, was captured at Salerno and held prisoner for sixteen months. Others in the group of P.O.W.s included veterans of fighting in France and

Italy, many of whom had been wounded before their capture. Technical Sergeant Len J. Hudgeons, who was shot in the stomach by a sniper, lay wounded for two weeks before being picked up by a German patrol and taken to Stalag 5-D. Hudgeons, a former instructor at Camp Hood, called out to German soldiers who saw he was wounded and carried him to their lines. Hudgeons survived in the field by giving himself morphine injections and by eating K-rations and raw turnip greens. Two Texans met in a Stalag hospital in Mantova, Italy. Sergeant Billy E. Radican of Mt. Vernon and Corporal James Roberts of Andrews were both wounded in Italy. Private First Class Ernest S. Harwell of Abbott was thrilled when he emerged from the train and found an old friend, Corporal Jesse Devers of West, who was an ambulance driver at McCloskey. Harwell was in a pillbox hit by a shell, and when he regained consciousness, found that his left foot had been blown off. The other Texans in the group were 2nd Lieutenant John Akers (Greenville, TX.), 2nd Lieutenant Finis A. Brumbeloe (Midlothian, TX.), 2nd Lieutenant Ernest Davis (Dallas, TX.), 2nd Lieutenant Ralph Norsworthy (Dallas, TX.), Technical Sergeant Eugene C. Damrel (Call, TX.), Private First Class Hobert C. Hunt (Florence, TX.), Technical Sergeant Travis G. Keeling (Avery, TX.), 2nd Lieutenant Elmer S. Proctor (Port Arthur, TX.), Private R. R. Lewellen (Mt. Pleasant, TX.), Staff Sergeant James H. Lawrence (Rusk, TX.), Private First Class Willie Martinez (Goliad, TX.), and Sergeant Jewel W. Phillips (Alto, TX.).[297] A group of new arrivals at McCloskey told of being pursued by German soldiers before making it back to their company. Technical Sergeant George Walton Daugherty of Imperial and Technician Fourth Grade Doyle (Dick) Daniel of Sweetwater felt lucky to be alive. Daniel, a company aid man in the 90th Infantry Division, was wounded twice while trying to help others. Daugherty, serving in Patton's 3rd Army, was hit by shrapnel in the head while on reconnaissance patrol.

Prisoners from Bilibid prisoner-of-war camp in the Philippines were treated at McCloskey General Hospital. Captain John B. Smith, a veteran of Bataan, told of the dire conditions at the prison where as many as 2,500 prisoners were confined to an area about 300 yards by 150 yards. Bilibid was a clearinghouse for all war prisoners in the Philippines. The "imperial food" consisted of a scant amount of rice and was supplemented only by a quarter of a caribou on the emperor's birthday. Smith said, "Our entire thoughts were of food." Captain Smith, who received a machine gun wound in the right leg, lost 55 pounds while interned for three years.[298] Another prisoner of war who survived Japanese imprisonment in the Philippines was Lieutenant Ruby F. Motley of Columbia, Missouri. Motley arrived at McCloskey in October 1945 to become the head dietitian after spending three years in Santo Tomas, a civilian prison. In prison, Motley oversaw the children's kitchen during her first year. Prisoners were never granted any freedom, but civilian Filipinos risked their lives throwing bags over the walls and smuggling newspapers into the camp. According to Motley, it was during their last year of imprisonment that the internees really suffered. Four men who helped smuggle money into the camp were caught and sent to a Japanese torture camp. Subsequent press releases indicated they were shot.[299] Several members of the Lost Battalion, the 131st Field Artillery, received medical care at McCloskey after surviving Japanese prison camps. Corporal Denzil O. Shores of Abilene, Corporal Herbert R. Morris of Cisco, and Sergeant Earl F. Baldock of Big Spring compared their experiences of being beaten with bullwhips and eating snails and cat and dog meat.[300]

What the Japanese could not do to one man, baseball did. Lieutenant John V. Lindsey of Moody, Texas, was a bombardier with 31 missions over targets in the South Pacific to his credit. Lindsey, an avid baseball player, promoted the sport between missions. He organized teams and carved out fields in the jungles of Guadalcanal, the Admiralties, Wadke, Noemfoor, and Morotal. At Morotal Airfield, the lieutenant was playing third base in a softball game and was shot in the arm before he realized it. His injury required extensive treatment not available overseas, so he was sent to McCloskey to recuperate.[301]

There were many stories of wounded soldiers and their long road back to health. Sergeant James Thomas Good of

Cache, Oklahoma, was the recipient of a steel plate in his skull to repair damage done by a bomb fragment as he repaired a transport plane on the Burma supply route in India. Unconscious for two weeks, he was transported to the States via a freighter, a trip that took 78 days. Brain surgeons assured him that with new techniques and metal discoveries for patching skull wounds that his head would look normal in a few months.[302] Private George Nelson of Crisfield, Maryland, was among the reconnaissance group that first landed on the Japanese-held island of Attu in May 1944. Some of the men were trapped in the snow and ice, went to sleep and never awoke. Nelson managed to stay awake and return to his ship seven days later, but his feet were black and frozen as hard as blocks of ice. Both feet were amputated at Letterman General Hospital in San Francisco. Nelson came to McCloskey in August 1944 where his legs were re-amputated, and the stumps were shaped and toughened with exercise as they healed. In December he was fitted with artificial legs, and by the end of March, he was walking naturally and ready to go home. Nelson's prosthetic legs were like the hundreds of others fitted to other amputees. The wooden feet were notched at the toe and hinged together with rubber filling so that movements looked normal. A rubber pad, placed under the heels, provided a natural bounce. Each soldier was fitted individually to mimic his own steps and gait. Another McCloskey patient wounded at the battle of Attu was a bit out of the ordinary. Private WAAC, serial number K-9999, was hospitalized along with her human comrades. A small white dog from California, WAAC was wounded on her left side by a piece of shrapnel. When it was suggested that she remain at Letterman General Hospital in San Francisco to recuperate, her buddies, who were headed to McCloskey, protested, and she was permitted to accompany them, riding first class in a Pullman car.[303] As they say, "Every dog has its day!"

Although combat injuries were most common, not all accidents occurred overseas as Staff Sergeant William C. Clifford of Camden, New Jersey attested. He was working on the motor of an M-10 tank destroyer at Camp Polk, Louisiana, when his hand caught and was torn off. Corporal Raymond P. Hamilton of Clide, Kansas, was one of many who lost arms in combat. The improvements in prosthetic arms since the first World War enabled men to learn to use their hands normally, and Hamilton was pictured operating a movie projector and Clifford demonstrating the use of his mechanical hand.[304] Sergeant Elmer Jay Morris of Ringling, Oklahoma, lost parts of three limbs, an eye and a finger in the Battle of the Bulge. Serving with the 35th Division, Morris and his fellow soldiers were trapped in a house when a German tank fired through the window, badly injuring him. As a prisoner, he received meager medical care and the Germans amputated both legs. In Morris' hometown, an "Elmer Chest" sponsored by the Rotary Club and the American Legion was on display in a local store to receive money for a trust fund established for the couple. His photo and story were picked up by many newspapers across the nation, showing Morris sitting in a wheelchair alongside his wife, Velma Lee. The smiling couple were "looking forward cheerfully to a chicken farm and happy future back home."[305] Not all stories had happy endings. One war hero and recipient of the Silver Star, the Bronze Star, and the Purple Heart, Corporal Stanley Heck, found that his wife had been unfaithful to him while he was overseas. His legs were blown off and one arm mangled when he stepped on a German land mine, but he said the actions of his wife were "the most painful hurt of all."[306] Hospitalized at McCloskey, Heck was unable to appear in court, but two lawsuits were filed on his behalf.

Elmer Morris was just one of many patients encountered by Gloria H. Cowan, a medical secretary at McCloskey from 1944 to 1945. She was employed there for thirteen months while her husband recovered from injuries sustained during the war. Gloria was born in New York City in 1922. She met Milton H. Cowan in 1939 at the New York World's Fair, and they married in 1942 while Milton was a Cadet at Clemson. He served in the army and was wounded by sniper-fire while fighting in France. He spent over a year recovering at McCloskey Hospital, including surgery to repair nerve damage, never fully successful. In 1946, after leaving Texas and returning to New York with her husband, Gloria received letters from several of the soldiers she met while at McCloskey and read newspaper and magazine articles about these young men who had sacrificed so much. The letters and articles prompted her to write about these heroes and their bravery. The following version of Gloria's story includes the letters and news articles she saved and retains her original writing with minor additions, editing, reorganization and captions by her daughter, Susan Claire Kimball of Lexington, Virginia.

GOODBYE, SECRETARY, GOODBYE!
By Gloria H. Cowan

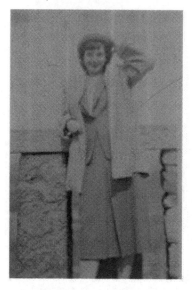

    The first letter came not long after my return from Texas in 1945. I couldn't have been more excited than if I had received my first love letter. Red-headed Clifford Leach, who had limited use of his arms and knew he must live the rest of his life in a wheelchair, had written a letter. It began:

Helo Gloria how are you doin

Very fine I hope
well I am doin all rite
now I on a amption ward…

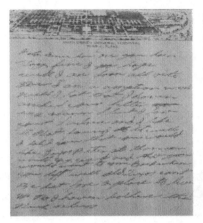 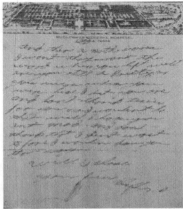

	2
Helo Gloria how are you doin	and then another nurse
Very fine I hope	I wont they ran the
well I am doin all rite	ward when you left well
now. I an a amption ward	are you still a Pretty as
Well I hat that I haven	you were when you
answered your letter	were here I bet you are
any sooner I but I lost	and don't think teasin
your address and I like	for you no I wouldnt do
to not found it. well	that well I hope you
I told you that you would	ant mad and don't
like Texas beter at than you	think that I don't want
would New York and that you	to fore I wouldn do you
would want to come back when	that way.
you left well old Texas cant	Well I close
Be bet fore a place to live.	Your fren Clifford
No I haven bothere the	
New secretary	

When my husband returned home from work that evening, I showed the letter to him and, forgetting about dinner, we began to talk about Clifford and the other boys we had met during the thirteen months we had spent at McCloskey General Hospital in Temple, Texas, where Milt had been a patient, and I a medical secretary. Once again, I was back on ward 20B and Cliff Leach, whose chart read he was six feet two inches tall, was wheeling himself into my office. One glance at that blaze of red hair and the look of mischief in his blue eyes and I knew I was in for much teasing. Lieutenant Harkins, our ward nurse, told Leach he was to stay out of her office and gave him permission to plague me instead. And plague me he did! Leach was an unusual patient for he had not lost any limbs. He had been completely paralyzed at first, but after two operations, with more to come, had regained partial use of his arms. His legs were lifeless, and the doctors agreed he would never walk again. In his wheelchair he looked small and shrunken, his body making a strange contrast to his arms, which hung abnormally long over the sides of his chair. "Old Leach must be improving if he can write now" Milt remarked, and then added "I hope they'll be able to do something for him to enable him to walk again. After all, I was totally paralyzed for a while." "Yes," I replied, "but you were more fortunate. Yours was a nerve injury and could be repaired, but his is spinal." "He sure was a devil, wasn't he? I'll never forget the day I was waiting for you outside of the office when he and Claude Dill passed by me, talking about you. They didn't know who I was and so when I asked them what they thought of the new secretary, Leach said "soooome babe" and Dill whistled. Weren't they the embarrassed fellows when you introduced me to them later on?" We laughed and laughed, remembering the boys' good humor. Aside from women, Leach's other interest was food. When the kitchen orderlies raced through the corridors pushing their bright chromium trucks with the trays piled high on them, Leach's face lit up. Those were the only times that he would leave my office and head cheerfully for his own room. Although he was in many ways worse off than the other boys in the ward who would one day wear artificial limbs and move about with ease, Leach was full of fun. He never talked about his past or his future, never mentioned his combat experience, never complained about his helplessness.

As Milt and I reminisced, it seemed that those weeks and months at the hospital had all been pleasant. We forgot the uncomfortable Texas heat, and only remembered the fun we'd had at the pool, the pride of McCloskey. We dismissed the image of a patient leaving his wheelchair at the rear of the movie house and painfully making his way to a seat, using his arms to help him move his body, and thought only of the humorous remarks the boys made while watching the movie. We even forgot the bitterness of our feelings as we watched the German prisoners of war in their enclosure near the hospital, playing baseball or eyeing the girls who occasionally passed.

My first day in the ward was something I shall never forget. Every boy who could hobble on crutches or wheel himself came to the office to meet me. Most of them brought hamburgers and cokes, and I began to wish I had a manual on how to eat dozens of hamburgers and keep smiling. Sixty in all, the boys thought they would be more welcome if bearing food. I couldn't refuse their gifts, nor could I thank each boy, dismiss him, and hope to hide that hamburger in my desk drawer. Each boy remained to see how much I enjoyed his friendship offering. So, I ate hamburgers, swallowed cokes and we were buddies. After that first day, the boys would bring anything they could find or steal: a jar of tomato juice, gardenias from the General's private garden, thermometers, pencils, playing cards and even dice. A steady stream of wheelchairs rolled in and out of the office each day. The boys came on any pretext: to ask for a furlough they knew they couldn't have, or to inquire for the doctor, having seen him leave. Captain Parker, our ward doctor, found he could seldom get into the office without stumbling over the crutches or pushing aside wheelchairs. He finally issued orders that patients could only visit the office if on official business. I was never sure, but I thought I heard him mutter on the day the order was posted on the door "you're a fire hazard." Official orders kept most of the boys out of the office, but not Leach. He was well named.

After a week I felt as though I had always lived in a world populated by men who had stumps instead of legs, flaps of skin in place of an arm or a hook rather than a hand. To my amazement, the boys were unaware of their plight, or so it seemed. They discussed their disabilities in terms of pension; the "hundred percenter" was envied despite his total disability.

182

Occasionally, I heard about a girlfriend breaking her engagement to a boy who had lost his leg or arm, but this was rare. The boys lived in a world of their own where all were handicapped.

They visited the occupational therapy shop, casually throwing a stump over the arm of a wheelchair, and relaxed and gossiped while working on leather belts or pocketbooks. But on Mondays, the day for ward rounds, when they looked down at the unbandaged wrecks of their bodies, they faced reality. As Captain Parker examined each patient, exposing the raw stump of an arm or leg, each boy suddenly became quiet and tense. Gazing at his body, he again suffered his inexorable loss. In the silence of the room I could hear the thoughts of those boys as they realized that one day, they must leave the false security of the hospital and become part of the world outside where most men had two legs and two arms. There were no jokes on Mondays. After Captain Parker completed rounds, I would return to my office and type the progress notes without interruption; the boys did not visit me after Monday rounds. They were sitting or lying on their beds, reading and writing letters to the people they dreaded meeting again. But Leach never seemed despondent. He wore a shrug-of-the-shoulder look constantly, and after rounds his attitude was even more indifferent.

Claude Dill had the sweetest smile I had ever seen. He had been on the ward longer than most of my patients and had received his artificial limb. He had lost a leg during the Battle of the Bulge in Belgium, and the other foot had been damaged. It had not been determined while he was at McCloskey whether he would have to lose the other leg as well, or if his foot could be repaired in any way. Claude's letter arrived shortly after Leach's. He had been relocated to the U.S. Army's largest convalescent facility, Wakeman General Hospital at Camp Atterbury, Indiana. Claude had been in the same division as Milt, though a different company. A friendly rivalry sprang up between us as to which company had won the war in Europe.

We soon called each other "G Company" or "B Company." Accordingly, Claude's letter began: "Hello B Co."

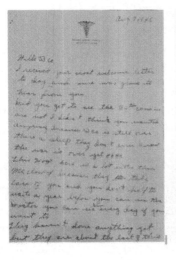

August 7 1945	
Hello B Co.. I received your most welcome letter to day and sure was glad to hear from you. Did you see the 30th come in are not I didn't think you wanted anyway because B Co. is still over there a sleep they don't even know the war is over yet HAHA. This Hosp. here is a lot better then McCloskey because they take care of you and you don't half to waite a year before you can see the Doctor you can see him every day if you want to. They haven't done anything yet but they are about the last of this	week and I'm realy glad because I've been waiting long enough for some thing to be done. I went on a three day pass this week end and what a time I had. I sure miss you and the time here gose so slow no one to talk to and kid around like I could you because they can't take it it's alright for them to kid you but when you kid them it all wrong. Tell your husband I said hello and be good and he'd better go over there and wake his Co. up so they can come back home. I wrote all I can think of so I'll say so long for now I was realy glad to get your letter and I will every one you so write as offen as you like because I'll always be more then glad to hear from you By now B Co. Sincerely, Claude Dill INDIANA

Claude was such a friendly chap. He spent long hours telling me of his home in Indiana, and his girl who was also named Gloria. He was delighted at the coincidence. He was nineteen and had spent most of those years on a farm. He had no plans but concentrated all his energy on trying to use his foot, hoping it could be saved. It was both wonderful and heartbreaking to hear him clumping down the halls, practicing. How thrilled he was whenever I told him he was improving.

One of Claude's good friends was Ralph Neppel. Ralph had lost both legs above the knee. Soon after he came to McCloskey, Ralph's fiancée, Jean, came from Iowa to be with him. She remained for a year while his wounds healed, and he learned to use his artificial limbs. Ralph was the hero of the ward and hospital. He endeared himself to everyone, nurses, doctors, fellow patients. He was more than liked; he was adored. Ralph was one of those rare people who live for others, considering everyone's comfort before his own, cheering other boys when perhaps he needed cheering himself, and sharing with all, whatever was his. In September 1945 Ralph Neppel was awarded the Congressional Medal of Honor in a ceremony held at The White House. I learned about it from an article in *Life Magazine*, never from Ralph himself. On December 14, 1944 Ralph was the leader of a machine gun squad situated on an approach to the village of Birgel, Germany when an enemy tank fired a high-velocity shell wounding his entire squad. Ralph was blown ten yards from his gun, had one leg severed below the knee and suffered other wounds, including damage to his remaining leg. He dragged himself back to his position on his elbows, remounted his gun and killed the enemy infantrymen accompanying the tank, forcing it to retreat. The devotion of Ralph's many friends in the ward was proven when Ralph had his legs re-amputated. He asked for and secured permission to have a re-amputation performed on both his legs at the same time. On the day he went into surgery I took the morning off and didn't report for work until he had been returned to his room. I found the ward in an uproar. Wheelchairs raced through the long corridors. Groups of angry patients stood together making angry gestures with their crutches and canes. I asked Claude Dill what happened. He was so angry that he stuttered when he replied. "They've gone and done a re-amp, on only one leg!" Cliff Leach added "Poor Ralph like to cried when he woke and found out about it." Jose Olvera, complainer in chief of the ward was all for demanding an official explanation. Just then, General Bethea, commander of the hospital and former battlefield surgeon, appeared on the ward. The boys became quiet when they saw their commanding officer, but their faces looked sullen. General Bethea was well-liked and respected. It was well-known that he had the welfare of his patients at heart. In this hospital an officer was, in a sense, at the mercy of a patient, for a complaint lodged against him brought the disapproval of General Bethea. "Boys" said the General, "the surgeons decided that Ralph couldn't stand the additional anesthesia required if both legs were re-amputated. They feared that Ralph would go into a state of shock. You can understand that can't you? It is better for Ralph to wait a few months longer rather than risk complications." The boys nodded in agreement with the General, but when he left Claude shouted: "you'd a thought they'd know before and not let Ralph expect them to do both legs!" Everyone trooped into Ralph's room where Jean was sitting beside his bed. Ralph tried to be cheerful. He and Jean had planned to get married on the day he could walk again, and now that meant a delay of many months. Every boy experienced the disappointment Ralph must be feeling.   A year and a half after Ralph had his second amputation, I ran across his picture in *Life Magazine*. Tall and handsome, Ralph stood beside his wife, Jean. Mr. and Mrs. Neppel could have been any normal couple. Who would have guessed the heroic struggle they had survived?

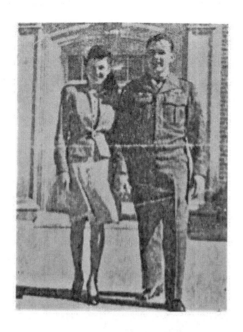

Looking at the photograph, I felt that Ralph would surely find his place in the world again. His fellow Iowans had presented him with a ranch-style house in Carroll, Iowa; the government provided him with a specially equipped automobile. And on November 28, 1948, four years after he lost his legs, *The New York Times* reported that 25-year old Ralph Neppel had harvested a 120-acre corn crop, double that which would normally be expected. He operated his own tractor and plowed by himself, producing a crop of 100 bushels per acre. Ralph's only complaint to the Veteran's Administration is that he wears out his artificial limbs too fast. Ralph had indeed made a place for himself.

Time in the hospital passed swiftly. Anything new, a movie, a visiting celebrity, a present from home, a new secretary in the next ward, or the arrival of a boy's parents, became exciting events. The day Elmer Morris' parents arrived at the hospital remains clearly impressed in my memory. Nineteen years old, Elmer Morris had lost his right arm and his right eye in combat. He had been taken prisoner by the Germans, his shoes taken from him and paper "shoes" substituted. In the terrible cold of that winter of 1944, Elmer's feet froze. An American doctor might have saved them, but the Germans amputated both legs. Elmer's parents and his girlfriend, Velma, came to the office, and I took them to his room. I dreaded the moment when they saw their son. But I had no reason to fear the meeting. There were no tears; Velma hugged and kissed her fiancée as though nothing had changed. Later, as I passed through the ward, they were happily talking and chatting about the folks back home. There was no strain. They were pretending nothing. They were glad to have Elmer with them again. The sight of those valiant people unnerved me for the first time since I came to the hospital, and back in my office I wept in helpless anger at the utterly useless destruction of war. But Elmer and Velma had such optimism for their future together. They married while he was still at McCloskey Hospital. The newspaper article I saved read that they were looking forward to starting a chicken farm and a happy future.

Not all parental visits made me sad. There was Jose Olvera. He was small in stature, had a dark complexion, and a beguiling innocent face that belied his devilish nature. He had lost his left leg below the knee and never ceased to remind everyone that he was a wounded hero.

Olvera's constant complaints were almost taken for granted on the ward. Our poor nurse, Lieutenant Hansen could hardly ever manage to get Olvera out of bed. Because she was constantly nagging him, he nicknamed her "Gravel Gertie" and she became known as "Gravel" to everyone. Ironically, Olvera finally did get something to complain about. He became jaundiced and was removed to the jaundice ward. I visited him most every day, and he seemed to be the yellowest patient on the ward. Olvera's letter arrived a week or so after Dill's. The first surprise was his beautiful handwriting, but then I remembered that he had graduated high school and had entertained ideas of going to college. It was all of three pages long. Reading his letter reflected complaints about his new diet.

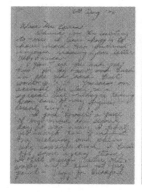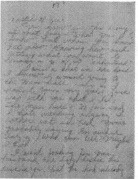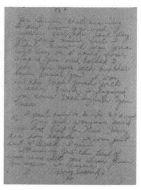

6th Aug '45	pg. 2	pg. 3
Dear Mrs. Cowan: Thank you for writing to me. I was happy to have heard from you and enjoyed reading your letter very much. How are you and your hub? I'm O.K. now and back in the old ward, but won't go to the barracks on account I'm still on a special diet — they're taking good care of my figure — aren't they? I gave "Gravel" a piece of my mind the second day I was here. I didn't get enough for breakfast one morning and when she came around I blew off some excess steam. I felt much better afterwards and I also got my point — 2 eggs for breakfast	instead of one. You know in this army it's not only — "what you know but whom you know" but also "knowing how and getting what you want" to make a go of it. Understand? I wts a shot in the dark. I knew I wasn't going to the mess hall even if I hadn't gain my goal. Luck was with me that I did. The mess hall's too far and I hate walking anyway. I rather eat in bed. You're probably saying I'm awful lazy. Who can tell? Maybe I am. I went looking for your husband the day before his discharge but he had already	for Temple that evening. I also saw you and another girl the last day you came over but I didn't know it was your last day or I would have stopped you and talked to you. You were with another dame weren't you? I was in the back porch with another friend. I figured you come back again. You never. I went over to Wards 20A and B. Some old woman said you had left for New Jersey the day before. I was just out of luck I guess. Wishing you the best of luck and let me hear from you again. I remain Very Sincerely, Jose

    While Olvera was ill, his huge family came from Missouri to see him. He had a little fat mother, a little fat father, and an odd assortment of nine sisters and brothers. They sat around his bed, gazing curiously and jabbering about the nurses, doctors and other patients, more interested in everybody except Jose. No wonder, I thought, that he demands attention; he must never have received any at home. His yellow face concerned the family more than his lost leg, but his younger brothers and sisters couldn't help giggling at him and all the boys with similarly yellow faces In the surrounding beds. Olvera's remark in his letter about not saying goodbye recalled that memorable day when Milt was discharged from the Army and we left the hospital. During my last day on the ward, my boys kept coming to the office to say goodbye. I made the rounds of all the bed patients whose shouts of "good luck" could be heard echoing down the halls. Suddenly my ward was empty of wheelchairs and patients on crutches. I presumed they were at a movie, so I started down the corridor, heading for the main exit. Like a wounded soldier, I was eager to return to civilian life yet experienced the sadness at leaving the security of the hospital. Here there were no housing or food problems. Who knew what might lie ahead? As I approached the exit, I saw that the hallway was lined with the boys on my ward. They formed a line on either side of the corridor and held out their canes and crutches, forming an archway over my head. I ran through that archway, tears welling up in my eyes, scarcely hearing their shouts:

"SO LONG, NEW YORK!"
"BE GOOD!"
"WRITE TO US!"
"LOTS OF LUCK!"
"GOODBYE, SECRETARY, GOODBYE!"

Chapter 12: The Fight Is Well Worth It

During an inspection tour of army hospitals in the Eighth Service Command in October 1945, Major General Norman T. Kirk announced the army's plans to close certain general hospitals. Speaking in Temple, Kirk said battle casualties reached their peak in August with 320,000 patients, and the numbers would continue to decline. He gave no indication which hospitals would be closed but declared the Brooke General Hospital in San Antonio, William Beaumont General Hospital in El Paso, and the Army-Navy Hospital in Hot Springs, Arkansas, would remain open. He hinted that the Veterans Administration would assume operation of closed hospitals although he said most of the hospitals built in the Eighth Service Command were not built for such a purpose.

In January 1946, General Omar Bradley, who had been appointed to head the Veterans Administration after the war, testified before a congressional appropriations sub-committee regarding the possible retention of McCloskey General Hospital and Ashburn General Hospital in McKinney by the V.A. The V.A. surveyed existing hospitals, and although many were found unsuitable, the "fine McCloskey plant [was] suitable for its needs." [307] The Veterans Administration requested 15 million dollars for construction of new, permanent, hospital buildings, but many believed existing facilities should be used whenever feasible. Construction of new buildings would take time and structures would not be ready for a year. An additional concern was recruiting a staff of doctors, nurses, technicians, and attendants needed to operate new hospitals. Using existing facilities would ensure that personnel would most likely stay on if operations were continuous whereas they would leave service or move into the private sector if their jobs were terminated or interrupted. The previous December, the V.A. was down 2,100 physicians and surgeons and 700 were on loan from the army. Recruitment efforts were underway to secure additional medical staff.

On March 31, 1946, McCloskey General Hospital closed. Over 100 patients who were still under physicians' care were transferred to other hospitals. The last patient was Arnold F. Witt, a 20-year-old amputee from Harvard, Illinois, who had served with the 517th Parachute Regimental Combat Team and lost his leg at Bastogne during the Battle of the Bulge. The Waco annex closed on January 5, 1946, with all remaining patients being picked up by the main hospital when they returned from Christmas furlough.[308]

A farewell dinner and dance were held for General Bethea, twelve officers, and two enlisted men who were departing for Fort Sam Houston where Bethea was to assume command of Brooke Army Hospital. Bethea said, "I have never left a post I hated to leave as much as I do Temple." He summed up his time in Temple:

> When I was in Temple, I was head of the biggest business there. Our payroll at McCloskey was over a million dollars a month at its height. We had joint medical meeting with the local doctors and our relations with them were perfect. I had warm friends at both the Scott-White Hospital and the King's daughters, as well as the Santa Fe. When we closed McCloskey Hospital and Margaret and I were leaving Temple, the people must have been glad to see us go. Besides the usual military farewell parties, the white civilian employees gave us a banquet. The Negro civilian employees gave us a banquet. The businessmen of Temple gave us a banquet and presented me with a beautiful watch. The Temple Post of the American Legion made me a life member. The Temple Rotary Club made me a lifetime honorary member, etc.[309]

Winnie W. Wynne wrote a poem entitled *"Our McCloskey"* to honor the hospital and General Bethea:

The time has come for us to say,
Farewell! McCloskey, on this sad day.
Not one of us will e'er forget
Those we love, and friends we've met.

McCloskey to us is not just a name,
It's a symbol for those who live again,
She's tenderly cared for the wounded and worn,
Through loving care they've been re-born.

She received her own by plane and rail
The boys who're back from a living hell.
With patience and skill, and nursing care,
New life for those both here and there.

Her beautiful grounds, with blooming flowers,
Helped many patients through long, long hours.
It helped their morale, for there to see,
Was the wonderful land of their own country.

To General Bethea, who has given his best,
We give of our blessings, along with the rest.
He is generous, patient, loving and kind,
Our loss is a gain for the next in line.

With flag unfurled she waves goodbye
To her workers who stood faithfully by.
She will live in History, not only in name,
But for Glory, Honor, Duty, and Fame.

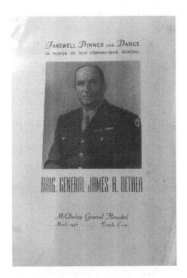

Farewell Dinner and Dance Program. SOURCE: Olin E. Teague Veterans' Center Medical Library Archives.

In April 1946, *The Austin American-Statesman* reported that "President Truman's approval has put the big McCloskey Army Hospital at Temple in the hands of the Veterans Administration and has restored it to service."[310] Five hundred beds at McCloskey would be used immediately on a temporary basis. A small staff assumed the task of organizing the hospital for V.A. use. Captain Albert F. Hart assumed command of McCloskey General Hospital, effective May 1, 1946. Lieutenant Colonel Joseph W. Westbrook of the Veterans Administration arrived in Temple to take over maintenance. Dr. L. M. Cochran, manager of the veterans' hospital in Amarillo, was transferred to Temple for 30-day temporary duty as head of the hospital in June. He was succeeded by Dr. Allan G. Fuller of Fort Bayard, New Mexico, to head the staff. Official word came from the Eighth Service Command headquarters, dated May 8, 1946,

Discontinuance of McCloskey General Hospital, Temple, Texas
1. Pursuant to authority in War Department letter, AB 602 (25 Feb 45) OB-I-SPMOC-M,

194

dated 28 February 1946, subject, "Surplus General Hospitals," McCloskey General Hospital was placed in the category of Surplus, effective 31 March 1946.

2. By authority of TWX, Headquarters, Army Service Forces, dated 1 May 1946, the accountability for and custody of subject installation was transferred to the Veterans Administration on 6 May 1946.

3. The 1884th Service Command Unit, McCloskey General Hospital, Temple, Texas, will be discontinued and Service Command Unit Number 1884 Withdrawn, effective 13 May 1946.
By command of Lieutenant General Walker
H.L. Boatner, Colonel, GSC, Acting Chief of Staff[311]

General Bradley made an inspection trip to Dallas in late 1946 where he conferred with a Texas delegation that included Congressman W. R. Poage, Temple's mayor Guy Draper, attorney Byron Skelton, newspaper publisher Frank Mayborn, and Myron Blalock of Marshall, Texas, national Democratic committeeman. Also, in attendance was Colonel Thomas G. Lanphier of Dallas, deputy V.A. administrator for the Southwest. The delegation reported that there were only 159 patients and 300 employees at McCloskey, and it proposed that part of the hospital campus be used to house the offices of other agencies such as the Department of Agriculture. Bradley stated that "taking over the Ashburn and McCloskey Army Hospitals at McKinney and Temple, Texas and LaGarde Hospital at New Orleans would alleviate the shortage of beds for veteran patients."[312] He promised a decision within two weeks on the future status of the hospital.

The Temple Daily Telegram reported on October 6, 1946, that high-ranking V.A. officials were in Temple for a dedication ceremony. Colonel Thomas G. Lanphier and Dr. Lee D. Cady, chief V.A. medical officer for Texas, Louisiana, and Mississippi, spoke of their vision of a first-rate Veterans Administration hospital in Temple with as many as 2,000 beds. Colonel Lanphier praised McCloskey as one of the finest general and surgical hospitals and disclosed plans that included housing and treating tubercular veterans there. Lanphier noted that Temple was the logical location for a V.A. hospital because of the medical expertise already present in the community.

In the meantime, a conflict erupted with representatives of the 11th District American Legion, Department of Texas, who insisted that the hospital be retained exclusively for Veterans Administration uses. The group convened in Waco in November 1946 to inform its members of telegrams sent by Commander Emmett Streetman to General Bradley, the Federal Board of Hospitalization, T. O. Kraabel (American Legion representative), Congressman Poage, and Colonel Lanphier:

> Many veterans now unable to get hospitalization; many men being held in service because veterans' administration is unable to furnish beds. Facilities at McCloskey are unexcelled for treatment of veteran patients. American Legion highly pleased with treatment now being received by veteran patients. Imperative that bed capacity be increased to maximum. Geographical location perfect for serving large center of population. Adequate transportation facilities to all sections of Texas. McCloskey Hospital located in great medical center which complies with Gen. Hawley's statement, "Hospitals should be located adjacent to large medical centers." A definite commitment to continue operation of McCloskey would be to

the best interest of the veterans of Texas. We will thank you for such a commitment.

Rumors were circulating that the V.A. planned to operate McCloskey as a tubercular center. Frank Mayborn told *The Austin American-Statesman* that "we told Bradley when in Washington that we had no objections to tubercular patients being housed at McCloskey, that our objection was in branding Temple as a tubercular center." Dr. Lee D. Cady responded that if McCloskey were not used, 800 tubercular patients in need of care would have to be treated elsewhere.

In 1947, Senator W. Lee O'Daniel questioned the V.A.'s decision to close McCloskey and construct other buildings in Marlin, home of Senator Tom Connally, and in Bonham, home of Congressman Sam Rayburn. In reply, Dr. Cady declined comment on Senator O'Daniel's statements and reminded the public that McCloskey had already been in operation for some time at about half the 1000-bed capacity. As part of his whistle-stop campaign for re-election in 1948, President Truman traveled by train across the state of Texas. Upon his arrival in San Marcos on September 27, he gave an informal train platform speech in which he mentioned McCloskey and its future:

> Now, I am told that this great city of Temple has a law on the books, which forces the President's train to stop whether he wants to or not. I want to say to you that I didn't know anything about that ordinance until I read a clipping from a Washington paper dated September 21. I was going to stop, anyway, so you didn't need an ordinance to get me to stop. Your Congressman says I promised to come here just before I took office way back there in January 1945. But it is most interesting, and I think I ought to read you this piece in this Washington paper: "It is a good thing that President Truman scheduled a

197

campaign stop in Temple, Tex." This is an Associated Press dispatch in the Washington Star. "The Marshal halted one Presidential train that was scheduled to pass through there without stopping. It's the law." I have heard for a long time about the excellent hospitals you have in this great city. This would be a fine place to recover from any illness. I have visited McCloskey Hospital during the war; it is one of the biggest Army hospitals in the land, and I hope we can continue to make use of it, because it is a fine plant."[313]

The situation dragged on until 1948 when Congressman Olin E. Teague proposed an inspection trip to the Midwest, Pacific coast, and Texas to obtain a current assessment of the needs of Veterans Administration hospitals. Teague told a reporter,

We want to know how well each of the existing facilities is serving the veterans in its area. If they are overcrowded, we want to know to what extent, and whether doctors and nurses will be available if they are enlarged. Veterans with service-connected disabilities certainly must get top priority. We want to be sure their needs are met, and then determine to what extent the VA hospitals can take care of other veterans.[314]

After conferring with Colonel Thomas G. Lanphier, head of the V.A.'s office in Dallas, Teague predicted that McCloskey would receive the increase in beds and expanded service that it had been seeking. He stated that likely patients also would be transferred from the hospital in Waco to alleviate congestion there.

McCloskey issued several appeals for nursing staff to meet the expansion of services to disabled veterans. Dr. L. M. Cochran addressed the shortage:

> I should like to emphasize the fact that our need for nurses here at McCloskey is really acute. Indeed, this is the major obstacle which is handicapping the expansion of our services to the disabled veteran. While we have been operating the hospital for a relatively short time, our waiting list is already large and growing daily. However, I believe that when the urgency of our situation is really understood by registered nurses in general, the response will be gratifying.
> [315]

Working conditions at McCloskey were lauded as well as the salaries for staff nurses. Nurses at McCloskey would have the opportunity of "pleasant surroundings with physicians and surgeons who are specialists in their fields and among the best in the nation." The annual salary for staff nurses began at $2,644.80 and $3,397.20 for supervisory positions. Nurses were furnished living quarters, subsistence, laundry and maid service for $40.00 per month. Assurances were given that for qualified applicants, the hiring process would proceed quickly to fill the numerous vacancies.

One such applicant was Helen Luco, a recent graduate of the cadet nurse program at Providence Hospital in Waco. She began her career at McCloskey on September 20, 1948, with a starting salary of $2,974. In addition to Helen, several graduates of the Providence nursing school applied at the hospital and arrived in Temple together: Margaret Sudduth (Hill), Aileen Hollas, Mildred Little, Ursula Trappe, and Verl and Grace (Campbell) Childers who had married during nurses' training at Providence. Helen lived on the hospital grounds in the barracks buildings which had been converted to nursing quarters. She later moved in with other nurses in a duplex apartment house on South 1st Street. In the beginning, they rotated to different wards, and Helen was eventually assigned to the orthopedics ward. Helen met her future husband, Aubrey Woolley, at the hospital where he was a nursing assistant on the orthopedics ward. They married in 1950. Her friend, Verl Childers, was head nurse of Ward 13B (the tuberculosis ward), and Mrs. Childers worked in the Intensive Care Unit.

In October 1949, a citizen committee composed of Frank Mayborn, Guy Draper, A.C. Scott, and Arthur Brashear went to Washington to meet with V.A. Chief, General Carl Gray, regarding the State of Texas' desire to use part of McCloskey Hospital as a state eleemosynary institution. The General assured the committee that McCloskey would not be forced to share space with any other veterans' hospital or state or federal agency. He informed them that the number of beds available in the state for veterans' care was below the national average, and he contemplated no change in the use of the hospital. McCloskey's current patient load was about 700 patients with a total capacity for 1,000. The domiciliary was activated on November 1, 1949, by a transfer of a member cadre from the centers at Biloxi, Mississippi; Thomasville, Georgia; and Wadsworth, Kansas.[316]

Temple citizens remained active in fighting for McCloskey's future as a veterans' hospital as other groups set their sights on the facility. In 1952 the U.S. Air Force announced plans to reactivate Moore Field in Mission where the Weaver H. Baker Sanitorium was quartered. The State Hospital Board approved construction of new tuberculosis units at Harlingen and San Antonio, but the patients had to be moved somewhere on a temporary basis before January 1, 1953. Governor Allan Shivers proposed moving 900 tuberculosis patients to the hospital and stated that "I personally am going to do everything I can to see that they get it (space in McCloskey)."[317] Resolutions against the governor's proposal were adopted by the Chamber of Commerce, American Legion, Disabled American Veterans, and the Optimist Club. Many other groups were expected to follow their lead. Veterans groups said they feared curtailment and deterioration of veterans' medical care if such a move was made. The Temple City Commission approved a resolution signed by Mayor Roy Strasburger stating they were "unalterably opposed" to Shivers' proposal. The City of Temple donated the land on which the hospital stood at a cost of $50,000 which the city was still paying on. Frank Mayborn, publisher of *The Temple Daily Telegram*, responded to the governor with a letter:

> Our fears of only "temporary use of McCloskey, while slightly soothed by your efforts to get two new hospitals activated for Latin-American TB's, are inspired by the long record of 'temporary' government facilities that have become permanent for reasons that they were not contemplated when the structures were erected or by the failure of promises that could not be kept because those who made them were no longer around to carry them out. [318]

Mayborn reminded the governor that three years earlier the city of Temple urged the legislature to locate a state surgical and general hospital at McCloskey. The request was rejected, and the funds were used for a hospital in Dallas. Mayborn added that only four buildings at McCloskey were available for use but had been offered to the Department of Agriculture by Representative Poage. He continued,

> Finally, you should know, as certainly your representatives in Washington today should learn, that there just isn't any space in McCloskey with which to solve your problem in the valley. If you continue to ruthlessly press your desire to have McCloskey for these unfortunate Latin-American tuberculars, we can only assume you prefer to put your state regional problems ahead of the war veterans. Seizing a portion of McCloskey isn't the solution to your problems,

Governor. It just can't be worked out in fairness to the veterans, Latin-Americans or Temple.[319]

The dispute only intensified when businessmen from three South Texas communities assailed Representative Poage. Poage joined the attack, declaring the Lower Rio Grande interests were based on business decisions related to the reactivation of Moore Field. The Tri-Cities Reactivation Committee, composed of businessmen from Edinburg, McAllen, and Mission, issued a statement saying the reactivation of Moore Field would save the federal government 23 million dollars. Meanwhile the mayor of Mission called Poage's statement a "damn lie" and turned the tables on him by accusing him of putting business interests ahead of sick people. Mayor Angus McLeod of McAllen went so far as to suggest that Poage and his constituents did not want Latin-American patients in Temple. [320] Poage responded with a letter to R. C. Tompkins, Executive Secretary of the Lower Rio Grande Valley Chamber of Commerce. In part, he said,

> Nowhere in Texas could the location of tubercular patients have a more disastrous effect. Temple provides the hospital facilities for a large part of Central Texas. The presence of these tubercular patients would effectively deny the people of the wide area the use of these facilities. It would be unfair to the civilian population. This would be cruel and ruthless as it involves the veterans who have no choice as to where they could go... Your letter refers to the interest of your people "in the humanitarian aspect of this matter." I believe that any serious concern for the humanitarian aspect would dictate that these unfortunate tuberculars should be kept as close as possible to their homes and loved ones. I have seen no evidence of any concern on the part of the

citizenship of South Texas for the unfortunate non-tubercular-- but equalled disabled veteran -- patients who now occupy a large part of McCloskey Hospital. The doctors of the V.A. have said that it would endanger the health and lives of the patients to put more tubercular patients in the institution.[321]

Eventually, all parties agreed to abide by the V.A.'s decision, but Mayborn was firm in his stance:

There is no room at McCloskey for 900 state TB patients or any other hospitalized group. Gov. Shivers' arithmetic is misleading. Subtracting the 1,000 beds in use now from the hospital's 3,100 capacity pictures McCloskey as a 1942 Army hospital. But not McCloskey as a 1952 VA hospital. [322]

In January 1953, the State of Texas acted on the tubercular patients from Weaver H. Baker hospital. Representative Joe Burkett, Jr. of Kerrville introduced a bill authorizing the State Hospital to transfer the patients to any other facilities it could acquire in Texas, and specifically to Legion Sanitorium which was part of the Veterans Administration hospital in Kerrville. Also requested in the bill was an appropriation for $100,000.00 for temporary rehabilitation of the Legion Sanitorium which had 350 available beds. Another 400 beds at a facility under construction in San Antonio would house the additional Valley patients until T.B. hospitals were built.

While officials were wrangling over the future of McCloskey and its use, a lawsuit was filed in the United States Court of Claims by the American Construction Company, the entity responsible for construction of the hospital. The War Contract Hardship Claims Act, also known as the Lucas Act, permitted recovery by war contractors on an equitable basis for losses resulting from war contracts if they could prove the losses arose without negligence or fault on their part. [323] The plaintiff entered into contracts with the War Department for the construction of McCloskey General Hospital at Temple, dated June 23, 1941, as well as the construction of Camp Normoyle in San Antonio, and Foster Field in Victoria. In the performance of the three contracts, the plaintiff sustained a net loss of $59,768.42 without fault or negligence. The loss on McCloskey Hospital was $73,727.74. During the performance of the contract, the construction company filed several written claims requesting reimbursement for expenditures covering a portion of premium time and excess costs caused by the actions of the Area Engineer. The construction company contended that it was required to increase the number of workmen and their hours of employment, but this did not accelerate the completion of the contract. Delays were caused by bad weather, and the extra costs incurred for additional labor could have been avoided. The claimant asserted that the Area Engineer was not "a practical construction man and was unduly influenced by his chief assistant, Mr. Dotson." The Area Engineer advised the claimant that "irrespective of what happened this job would be finished on contract time if within his power, that he was looking after his personal record and did not care if the claimant went broke."[324] On January 18, 1943, the plaintiff filed a written claim with the contracting officer for reimbursement of a portion of the overhead ($2,463.07) incurred in the construction of curbs and gutters. The claim was denied, and the plaintiff appealed to the Board of Contract Appeals. On November 25, 1944, the Board of Contract Appeals dismissed the appeal. What followed were years of continued efforts to obtain legal remedy. In due course, the plaintiff filed a petition in the Court of Claims on January 24, 1949. The court found in favor of the plaintiff and its ruling stated that

> "plaintiff is equitably entitled to the sum of $59,768.42 in settlement of its claim. Therefore, pursuant to Section 6 of the Lucas Act, *supra*, an

order will be entered directing the Department of the Army to settle such a claim in accordance with the findings of this court, in the amount of $59,768.42.[325]

Chapter 13: A Legacy of Excellence

When the war ended and the Veterans Administration inherited many of the hospitals built by the military, it soon discovered some hospitals were in obscure places and were expensive to operate. Some hospitals closed, and a large number needed improvement. The congressional Committee on Veterans' Affairs conducted an extensive survey of hospitals throughout the country in order to devise a program for modernization and replacement. Congressman Olin E. Teague of Texas headed the committee and released the survey results in March 1955. He stated, "The situation in many of our hospitals is acute."[326] Although many hospitals were built during the war, some 341 buildings were constructed prior to 1900. Teague and his colleagues in the Eighty-third Congress applied just enough pressure to gain President Eisenhower's recommendation for fifty-three million dollars for renovation and replacement of hospitals in his 1956 budget. During the Eisenhower administration, "Tiger" Teague's tenacity in the face of budget cuts and political machinations secured a victory for veterans everywhere. The president, in his 1960 budget message, said, "A first rate hospital and medical care program is also being provided. During the past year, a long-range policy for stabilizing the Veterans Administration hospital program at 125,000 beds has been established, and beginning with the 1961 budget, a twelve-year hospital modernization program is being initiated that will ultimately cost $900 million."[327]

Despite issues in many V.A. hospitals, the Temple center often received praise from congressmen and other officials and was cited for its efficiency in 1960. Statistics were released to demonstrate the hospital's efficiency. Since its transition in 1946, the hospital treated 51,841 patients. Additional statistics cited showed the Temple hospital with the fourth lowest per-day costs of 171 Veterans Administration installations around the country. The per-day cost in the hospital section during the previous fiscal year was $19.32 per patient and $3.55 per domiciliary member. The total cost of operating the hospital and domiciliary was $5,657,461. Salaries for 870 full-time and part-time employees and consultants totaled about 4.5 million dollars. The average daily hospital census was 700 patients and 385 domiciliary members. The dietetic service prepared 383,653 meals and special diets, and the housekeeping division cleaned and maintained 603,046 square feet of floor space.[328]

The Temple hospital received authorization for a new 10-million-dollar facility in 1958, and planning began during the Kennedy administration. The new Temple facility would consist of one single building to replace the 100 buildings constructed during the war. The site selected was in the approximate center of the hospital grounds, and the completion date was expected to be in June 1966. The new hospital was located only a mile or two from Scott and White Hospital's new 8-million-dollar building which was also under construction.

A groundbreaking ceremony was held November 11, 1964, at the construction site which was just south of the existing hospital. Ceremonies were sponsored by the Temple Chamber of Commerce, and many local officials were in attendance. Durward Howard and the Temple High School band presented a 15-minute concert to begin the program. Chaplain James S. Parks gave the invocation, and Center director Dr. S. J. Muirhead extended a welcome. Buster Brown of the Chamber introduced special guests. Ted Connell of Killeen, past commander of the Veterans of Foreign Wars, spoke briefly. Frank Mayborn introduced the main speaker, Congressman W.R. Poage. Following his speech, Congressman Poage broke ground with a chrome-plated shovel.

The new building was completed in December 1966. The first patient, Dr. Horace Wedemeyer, a service-connected disabled veteran from Georgetown, was accepted in April 1967. Dedication of the facility was held on June 17, 1967, with top Washington officials present, including William J. Driver, head of the Veterans Administration. The *Temple Daily Telegram* featured a *Temple VA Hospital Dedication Section* in its Saturday, June 17, 1967, paper. The front page editorial, entitled

207

Salute to McCloskey, summed up the community's sentiments about the hospital:

Temple welcomes today an impressive array of Veterans Administration officials, members of Congress and others who will join in getting the new VA hospital off to an auspicious start. We are delighted they can be here and help open a new chapter in the life of an institution which has so long been an important part of the Central Texas scene. The historical details of the VA Center, which most of us in this area simply call "McCloskey" from World War II days, are set forth elsewhere in this edition. What is more difficult to put into words, however, is the close kinship between hospital and community which goes back a quarter of a century. It began with McCloskey Army General Hospital and an outpouring of community sentiment and generosity for the patients brought directly here from the battlefield, many of them amputees. We did what we could to rebuild their spirit. We took their families into our homes when housing was short. And after the war, when McCloskey became a VA center, this sentiment did not die. Through the years hundreds of Central Texans have given thousands of hours of volunteer service for the veterans who were patients. The VA Center is important economically to us. But much more than that, the people who work there, the patients who are treated there-- they belong to and are an important part of our community life. So, our salute today is not so much to new facilities. Rather, it is to the people who run the VA Center and who will be able to do a better job because of the new hospital, and to the veterans who will benefit from their compassion, to the veterans who deserve the best   care the nation can give, and to the pride of an area in its relationship with a fine institution that the new VA Center should be dedicated today.

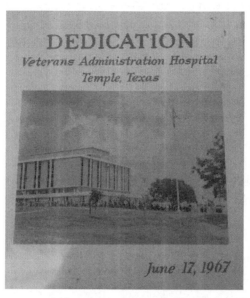

Dedication Day Program, 1967. SOURCE: Olin E. Teague Veterans' Center Medical Library Archives.

The new multi-story hospital contained 480 beds with cafeterias, stores, theater, and recreation facilities. Building 163 was a six-story, 240-bed general medical and surgical hospital with clinical facilities such as X-ray and laboratory for the entire hospital. Building 162 was a one-story 240-bed psychiatric hospital with eight 30-bed units. The psychiatric wards featured landscaped courtyards and lounge areas for television and recreation. Building 147 provided 7,000 square feet of floor space for medical research. A general and medical library supported reading and research interests of patients and physicians. More than 300 beds in portions of the old hospital were still in use, and the domiciliary had space for almost 400 patients, giving the hospital a total capacity of more than 1,000. Approximately 880 full-time employees were on staff, supplemented by volunteers from civic groups in the community.

The Temple domiciliary was one of only sixteen facilities operated by the Veterans Administration. The domiciliary environment provided a way to care for aging veterans who did not require acute hospitalization or skilled nursing services provided in nursing homes. Generally, eligibility for the domiciliary was based on the following needs: veterans requiring prolonged care in a sheltered setting or veterans with pressing medical needs or in need of intensive rehabilitation but who could return to the community following treatment. The Temple facility was considering the use of the domiciliary as a halfway house to prepare psychiatric patients prior to discharge.

The new hospital boasted up-to-date communications technology and equipment. Miles of tubing installed in the walls and forty-nine pneumatic tube sending and receiving stations provided a "30-second messenger service" for transmitting communications, drugs, or laboratory specimens. The transparent plastic canisters were 15 inches long and 5.5 inches in diameter with a pre-dialed brass ring to indicate the receiving station. Doctors were equipped with miniature electronic transistor receivers in their pockets, later known as "beepers." Intermittent beeps were transmitted and continued until the person being paged went to a telephone and called the operator to receive the message. Upon arrival at the hospital, doctors indicated their presence by flipping a switch on a registry board to let the hospital operator know they were on site and could be reached by phone or pager. The new hospital also contained a four-channel interhospital radio station. Connected to four commercial radio stations, the system could be dialed into any patient room.

Recreation continued to play a major role in the recuperation of the patients, and the *Temple Daily Telegram* compared the new V.A. Center amenities to those found at a summer resort rather than a government installation. Most of the facilities were built during its army hospital days-- the Olympic-size swimming pool, a nine-hole golf course and putting green, a gymnasium, bowling alley, and baseball-softball field. The greenhouse remained as a source of fresh flowers for the hospital.

With the building of the new high-rise hospital, many of the World War II-era buildings were torn down or declared surplus. By December 1967, Temple Junior College awaited word on the passage of a bill and a signature from President Lyndon B. Johnson on conveyance of 73 acres of land from the Temple Veterans Administration to the college. Public Law 90-197 was approved on December 14, 1967:

> Be it enacted by the Senate and House of Representatives of the United States of America in Congress assembled^ That the Administrator of Veterans' Affairs is authorized to convey, without monetary consideration, to Temple Junior College, Temple, Texas, for educational purposes, all right, title and interest of the United States in and to a tract of seventy-three acres of land, more or less, constituting a portion of the reservation of the Veterans' Administration Center, Temple, Texas. The exact legal description of the tract shall be determined by the Administrator of Veterans' Affairs, and if a survey is required in order to make such determination, the Temple Junior College shall bear the expense thereof. SEC. 2. Any deed of conveyance made pursuant to this Act shall— (a) provide that the land conveyed shall be used for educational purposes and in a manner that will not, in the judgment of the Administrator of Veterans' Affairs, or his designate, interfere with the care and treatment of patients in the Veterans' Administration Center, Temple, Texas; (b) contain such additional terms, conditions, reservations, easements and restrictions as may be determined by the Administrator of Veterans'

Affairs to be necessary to protect the interest of the United States (c) provide that if the Temple Junior College violates any provision of the deed of conveyance or alienates or attempts to alienate all or any part of the parcel so conveyed, title thereto shall revert to the United States; and that a determination by the Administrator of Veterans' Affairs of any such violation or alienation or attempted alienation shall be final and conclusive; and (4) provide that in the event of such reversion, all improvements made by Temple Junior College during its occupancy shall vest in the United States without payment of compensation there for. [329]

The 73 acres were part of the original acreage donated by the city of Temple for use in the construction of the army hospital and later transferred to the Veterans Administration. The swimming pool and golf course were jointly used by V.A. patients and T.J.C. students until such time that college expansion made operations impossible. Houses on the property formerly occupied by V.A. physicians were converted to faculty housing. Expenses assumed by the college were expected to be about $10,000 annually. The actual property transfer which tripled the size of the college did not take place until 1968. The college president, Dr. Hubert M. Dawson, said there were plans to put the property to immediate use with construction of a new $500,000 health and physical education building beginning in September 1968.

In 1978, Representative Ray Roberts of Texas introduced a bill in Congress to designate the Veterans Administration Center located in Temple as the "Olin E. Teague Veterans' Center." It became law on August 28, 1978 and took effect on January 4, 1979. Olin E. Teague, a war hero, was the most decorated U.S. combat soldier of World War II after Audie Murphy.[330] Teague spent two years recuperating in army hospitals, including McCloskey, after being wounded six times.

While at McCloskey, Colonel Teague asked to be made personal affairs officer in order to assist other veterans. He was known to make his way through the wards on crutches to talk with men about their problems. He assisted them with getting overdue promotions, settling family disputes, and solving financial issues.[331] He later served in Congress from 1946 to 1978 and was a relentless champion of veterans' affairs. In 1947, Teague himself had proposed a name change for McCloskey to "The 36th Division Memorial Veterans Hospital." Teague felt the designation was "particularly appropriate because the first large group of amputees to reach the Temple institution were 36th Division men wounded at Salerno in the Italian campaign."[332]

Both Camp Hood and McCloskey General Hospital brought great economic and social change to Temple and Bell County. Temple moved from a primarily agricultural area to a bustling hospital center. Throughout the war, Temple was often featured in new stories lauding the hospital and other war projects in the area. By February 1944, Temple's population had doubled to 30,000 people.[333] Only a few buildings of the original army hospital exist today. Most have been demolished and replaced with new structures. Later additions of a nursing home, domiciliary, satellite outpatient clinic, a 25-million-dollar clinical expansion, and partnership with Texas A&M University College of Medicine have resulted in the Olin E. Teague Veterans' Medical Center maintaining its vital role in the Central Texas community seventy years later.

Endnotes

Chapter 1

[1] Vivian Elizabeth Smyrl, "Temple, Texas," in *Handbook of Texas Online* (Texas State Historical Association, June 15, 2010), https://tshaonline.org/handbook/online/articles/hdt01.

[2] "History of Bell County Medical Alliance," Bell County Medical Alliance, January 2015, http://www.bellcountymedicalalliance.com/history.html.

[3] Odie B. Faulk and Laura E. Faulk, *Frank W. Mayborn: A Man Who Made a Difference* (Belton, TX: University of Mary Hardin-Baylor, 1989), 112.

[4] "It's a Cotton Christmas," *The Corpus Christi Caller-Times*, December 4, 1939, 4.

[5] *The Templar: Yearbook of Temple Junior College, 1939/1940* (Temple, TX: Temple Junior College, 1940), https://texashistory.unt.edu/ark:/67531/metapth979001/: accessed December 16, 2019), University of North Texas Libraries, The Portal to Texas History, https://texashistory.unt.edu, 14.

[6] Gerhard Peters and John T. Woolley, "Proclamation 2352—Proclaiming a National Emergency in Connection with the Observance, Safeguarding, and Enforcement of Neutrality and the Strengthening of the National Defense Within the Limits of Peace-Time Authorizations," The American Presidency Project, accessed February 18, 2019, https://www.presidency.ucsb.edu/node/210003.

[7] *Peace and War, United States Foreign Policy, 1931-1941*, United States. Department of State Publication 1983 (Washington, DC: Government Printing Office, 1943), https://hdl.handle.net/2027/mdp.39015023272209.

[8] "Americans and the Holocaust," United States Holocaust Memorial Museum, accessed February 29, 2020, https://exhibitions.ushmm.org/americans-and-the-holocaust/us-public-opinion-world-war-II-1939-1941.

[9] "Hitler Declares England Will Fall During New Year," *The Austin American-Statesman*, January 1, 1941, 2.

[10] "New U.S. Production Peak Is Due In 1941," *Temple Daily Telegram*, January 1, 1941, 1.

[11] Michael Kelsey, *Temple*, Images of America (Charleston, S.C.: Arcadia Publishing, 2010), 48.

[12] Clifford Joseph Hughes, "A Study of Temple, Texas During World War II" (Master's, Southwest Texas State University, 1972), 9.

[13] "'Bundles For Britain' Drive Has Successful Opening Day," *Temple Daily Telegram*, February 4, 1941, 1.

[14] "Defense Savings Bond Campaign Started Here," *Temple Daily Telegram*, May 2, 1941, 1.

[15] "Iron For Britain In Belton Grows," *Temple Daily Telegram*, May 1, 1941, 10.

[16] "Familiar Landmark, Old City Standpipe Torn Down For Scrap," *Temple Daily Telegram*, July 10, 1941, 1.

[17] "Pots and Pans Clatter Tune," *The Austin American-Statesman*, July 22, 1941, 1.

[18] "Temple's March of Pans Gets Splendid Start," *Temple Daily Telegram*, July 22, 1941, 1.

[19] "Parts of World War 1 Plane Added To Aluminum Pile Here," *Temple Daily Telegram*, July 25, 1941, 1.

[20] "Three-Ton Load of Aluminum Sent From Bell County," *Temple Daily Telegram*, August 3, 1941, 1.

[21] "New School Radio Series Opens Today," *Temple Daily Telegram*, February 4, 1941, 3.

[22] "Keep 'Em Flying Week Proclaimed by Mayor Mason," *Temple Daily Telegram*, August 19, 1941, 1.

[23] Franklin Delano Roosevelt, "Press Conference #762" (Executive Offices of the President, August 19, 1941), FDR Library, http://www.fdrlibrary.marist.edu/_resources/images/pc/pc0121.pdf.

[24] Patricia K. Benoit, "Backroads: Christmas Parade Is a Temple Tradition," *Temple Daily Telegram*, December 5, 2016,

https://www.tdtnews.com/news/article_aaf866d2-bab2-11e6-a9cf-9b27125843dd.html.

[25] United States Census Bureau, *1950 Census of Population: Volume 1. Number of Inhabitants. Texas* (Washington, DC: Government Printing Office, n.d.), https://www2.census.gov/library/publications/decennial/1950/population-volume-1/vol-01-46.pdf.

[26] Odie B. Faulk and Laura E. Faulk, *Frank W. Mayborn: A Man Who Made a Difference* (Belton, TX: University of Mary Hardin-Baylor, 1989), 114. A thorough account of Mayborn's life and civic contributions are enumerated in detail in this work.

[27] Ibid., 116.

[28] Ibid., 117.

[29] Ibid.

[30] Ibid., 119.

[31] Ibid., 121.

[32] Patricia K. Benoit, "Backroads: Santa Fe Hospital: 'A Delightful Place to Be Ill,'" *Temple Daily Telegram*, January 6, 2014, http://www.tdtnews.com/news/article_93929454-769a-11e3-adbf-001a4bcf6878.html.

[33] "Hospitals Bring Fame to Temple as Clinical, Surgical Center," *Temple Daily Telegram*, June 25, 1941, 9. The Woodson Hospital was housed with Scott and White but was a separate institution specializing in eye, ear, nose, and throat treatment.

[34] Faulk and Faulk, 122.

[35] Ibid.

[36] "Temple Given Multi-Million War Hospital," *The Clifton Record*, January 16, 1942, 1.

[37] "Army Base Hospital Awarded Temple," *Temple Daily Telegram*, January 7, 1942, 1.

[38] Faulk and Faulk, 129.

Chapter 2

[39] Kristy N Kamarck, "The Selective Service System and Draft Registration: Issues for Congress," *CRS Report* (Washington,

DC: Congressional Research Service, January 28, 2019), https://crsreports.congress.gov/product/pdf/R/R44452.

[40] Bernard D. Rostker, *Providing for the Casualties of War: The American Experience Through World War II* (Santa Monica, CA.: RAND, c2013), https://www.rand.org/pubs/monographs/MG1164.html, 176.

[41] Ibid, 177.

[42] Stephen E. Ambrose, *D-Day, June 6, 1944: The Climactic Battle of World War II* (New York: Simon & Schuster, 1994).

[43] Clarence McKittrick Smith, *The Medical Department: Hospitalization and Evacuation, Zone of Interior*, 1989 printing, United States Army in World War II: The Technical Services, CMH Pub. 10-7 (Washington, DC: United States Army. Center of Military History, 1956), 3.

[44] Rostker, *Providing for the Casualties of War: The American Experience Through World War II*, 217.

[45] Smith, 3.

[46] Ibid., 19.

[47] Ibid., 88.

[48] Ibid.

[49] Ibid., 14.

[50] Ibid., 23.

[51] Ibid.

[52] Lindsay Hannah, "United States Third Generation Veterans Hospitals, 1946-1958" (Washington, DC: National Park Service, Winter 2017), https://www.dot7.state.pa.us/CRGIS_Attachments/Survey/201 8M001042A_01H.pdf.

[53] Clarence McKittrick Smith, *The Medical Department: Hospitalization and Evacuation, Zone of Interior*, United States Army in World War II (Washington: Office of the Chief of Military History, Dept. of the Army, 1956), 77.

[54] Ibid., 68.

[55] Norman T. Kirk, "Memorandum for Control Division, Services of Supply," *Annual Report* (Surgeon General of the United States Army, August 18, 1942).

[56] Rostker, *Providing for the Casualties of War: The American Experience Through World War II,* 218.

[57] Leonard T. Peterson, "The Army Amputation Program," *The Journal of Bone and Joint Surgery* 26, no. 4 (October 1944): 635.

[58] Ibid.

[59] Rostker, *Providing for the Casualties of War: The American Experience Through World War II,* 219.

[60] Christina M. Barrett, *Dreeben-Irimia's Introduction to Physical Therapist Practice for Physical Therapist Assistants,* 3rd ed. (Burlington, MA: Jones and Bartlett, 2016), 13.

[61] Emma E. Vogel et al., "Training in World War II," in *Army Medical Specialist Corps*, AMEDD Corps History (Washington, DC: Department of the Army. Office of the Surgeon General; printed by Government Printing Office, 1968), https://history.amedd.army.mil/corps/medical_spec/chaptervi.html, 150.

[62] Ibid., 153.

[63] Ibid.

[64] Vogel et al., "Training in World War II", 159.

[65] Ibid., 160.

[66] Ibid., 163.

[67] "First Occupational Therapists Receive McClockey [sic] Diplomas," *Dallas Morning News*, June 24, 1945, 15.

[68] Emma E. Vogel et al., "Training in World War II," in *Army Medical Specialist Corps*, AMEDD Corps History (Washington, DC: Department of the Army. Office of the Surgeon General; printed by Government Printing Office, 1968), https://history.amedd.army.mil/corps/medical_spec/chaptervi.html, 148.

[69] Thelma A. Harman, "Professional Services of Dietitians, World War II," in *Army Medical Specialist Corps*, AMEDD Corps History (Washington, DC: Department of the Army. Office of the Surgeon General; printed by Government Printing Office, 1968), https://history.amedd.army.mil/corps/medical_spec/chaptervi.html, 187.

[70] Ibid., 191.

[71] Judith A. Bellafaire, *The Army Nurse Corps: A Commemoration of World War II Service*, Center of Military History Publication, CMH Pub 72-14 (U.S. Army Center of Military History, 2003), https://history.army.mil/books/wwii/72-14/72-14.HTM, 3.

[72] Office of War Information, *Information Program for the United States Cadet Nurse Corps* (Washington, DC: Government Printing Office, 1943), 9.

[73] Patricia K. Benoit, "Backroads: Nursing a Need: Cadet Corps Filled Shortage in World War II," *Temple Daily Telegram*, March 11, 2019, 3A.

[74] Bethea, "Annual Report of McCloskey General Hospital, Temple, Texas For the Calendar Year 1945," unpaged.

[75] "McCloskey Receives First Cadet Nurses," *Pampa Daily News*, June 23, 1944, sec. Back the Fifth, 2.

[76] *McCloskey General Hospital, Temple, Texas [Christmas Menu]* (S.l.: United States Army, 194?), unpaged.

[77] "Grave Shortage of Nurses in Army, Says Col. Zita Callaghan," *Belton Journal and Bell County Democrat*, December 28, 1944, 7.

[78] Charlotte R. Rodeman, *Neuropsychiatry in World War II. Pt. IV: Supporting Services and Personnel* (U.S. Army Medical Department. Office of Medical History., 2009), https://history.amedd.army.mil/booksdocs/wwii/NeuropsychiatryinWWIIVolI/DEFAULT.htm, 636.

[79] "8 Girls in Pinafores Delight in Aide Work at McCloskey," *The Austin American-Statesman*, May 21, 1944., 3.

Chapter 3

[80] "Army Base Hospital Awarded Temple," *Temple Daily Telegram*, January 7, 1942, 1.

[81] Hughes, "A Study of Temple, Texas During World War II", 45.

[82] Ibid., 46.

[83] Ibid., 43-44.

[84] Judith S. Cohen, "Pelich, Joseph Roman," in *Handbook of Texas Online* (Texas State Historical Association, June 15, 2010), http://www.tshaonline.org/handbook/online/articles/fpepv.

[85] "Army Hospital Work Started," *Temple Daily Telegram*, March 8, 1942, 1.

[86] "Army Hospital Construction Will Start Early April," *Temple Daily Telegram*, March 15, 1942, 1.

[87] Hughes, 48."

[88] James A. Bethea, *Memoirs of James A. Bethea* (San Antonio, TX.: Naylor Co, c1964), 101.

[89] Harry Blanding, "McCloskey Hospital One Building: Plant One of World's Largest," *Temple Daily Telegram*, November 4, 1942, 10.

[90] Hughes, "A Study of Temple, Texas During World War II", 47.

[91] "Draughon-Miller Central Texas Regional Airport | Temple, TX," City of Temple, accessed March 7, 2020, https://www.ci.temple.tx.us/88/Airport-Services. With the end of the war, the military declared the airfield to be in excess. It was turned over to the City of Temple, which closed Temple Municipal Airport, and renamed Temple Army Airfield "Draughon–Miller" in honor of two Temple fliers who had died in World War II.

[92] Hughes, "A Study of Temple, Texas During World War II", 33.

[93] Ibid., 26.

[94] Ibid., 27.

[95] Hill C. Gresham, "Many Problems Facing Temple Need Solution," *Temple Daily Telegram*, January 25, 1942, 4.

[96] F. B. Russell, "Belton Needs Building Material," *Belton Journal and Bell County Democrat*, January 21, 1943.

[97] Frank W. Mayborn, "Temple Area Designated As 'Private Housing Priority Locality': New Quota Due," *Temple Daily Telegram*, April 14, 1942, 1.

[98] Hughes, "A Study of Temple, Texas During World War II", 48.

[99] Ibid.

[100] "Four-C College Fall Term," *The Cameron Herald*, September 3, 1942.

[101] Schulze, Jr., *U.S. Army McCloskey General Hospital*, 3.

[102] Ibid., 13.

[103] ""The Going Is Hard, But the Fight Is Well Worth It, Major McCloskey Wrote in Last Letter Before He Was Killed," *Temple Daily Telegram*, November 4, 1942, 15.

[104] Schulze, Jr., *U.S. Army McCloskey General Hospital*, 29.

[105] "For Us, the Living," *The Rattler*, November 20, 1942, 2.

[106] Schulze, Jr., *U.S. Army McCloskey General Hospital*, 26.

[107] Walter R. Humphrey, "Thousands Of Civilians Join In Army's Dedication Of Hospital," *Temple Daily Telegram*, November 5, 1942, 1. A conflicting account is given in Schulze's book, "The widow of Major McCloskey, as well as his only son, did not come for the dedication. Mrs. McCloskey stated she could not go through further emotional upheaval and declined to come."

[108] Schulze, Jr., *U.S. Army McCloskey General Hospital*, 14.

[109] Ibid., 26.

[110] Hughes, "A Study of Temple, Texas During World War II", 50.

[111] Bethea, *Memoirs of James A. Bethea*, 101.

[112] "Warm Southwest Becomes Greatest Army Hospital and Convalescent Area," *Abilene Reporter-News*, April 9, 1944, 5.

[113] Bethea, *Memoirs of James A. Bethea*, 101.

[114] "McCloskey Hospital, Army's Largest, Observes First Anniversary," *Temple Daily Telegram*, November 4, 1943, 1.

[115] Ibid.

[116] Hughes, "A Study of Temple, Texas During World War II", 54.

[117] Schulze, Jr., *U.S. Army McCloskey General Hospital*, 15. According to Schulze, the painting hung in the Administrative Building from 1942-1946 and was shipped to the Army Medical Museum in Washington, D.C. It was later transferred to storage at the Army Medical Museum at Fort Sam Houston.

[118] "Portrait of Late Major McCloskey Given to Hospital.," *The Dallas Morning News*, November 7, 1944, 2. This story indicates the painting hung in post library no. 2.

[119] Hill C. Gresham, "Opening of Army Hospital Marks New Era In Growth of City of Temple," *Temple Daily Telegram*, November 4, 1942, 9.

Chapter 4

[120] Victor E. Schulze, Jr., *U.S. Army McCloskey General Hospital: 1942-1946, Temple, Texas* ([United States]: s.n, 1993?) 21.
[121] James A. Bethea, *Memoirs of James A. Bethea* (San Antonio, TX: Naylor Co, c1964) 99-100.
[122] Ibid.
[123] Schulze, Jr., *U.S. Army McCloskey General Hospital,* 23.
[124] Ibid., 24.
[125] "Principal Chief Nurse at Hospital Starting Her 25th Year of Service with Army," *Temple Daily Telegram*, November 4, 1942, 4.
[126] Schulze, Jr., *U.S. Army McCloskey General Hospital*, 24.
[127] James A. Bethea, *Memoirs of James A. Bethea* (San Antonio, TX.: Naylor Co, c1964), 103.
[128] Hughes, "A Study of Temple, Texas During World War II," 50.
[129] Schulze, Jr., *U.S. Army McCloskey General Hospital,* 25.
[130] James A. Bethea and Dorothy Bethea Ellis, *Memoirs of James A. Bethea* (San Antonio, TX: The Naylor Company, c1964) 102.
[131] James A. Bethea, "Annual Report of McCloskey General Hospital, Temple, Texas For the Calendar Year 1945" (Temple, TX: McCloskey General Hospital, January 1, 1946), 48.
[132] Clifford Joseph Hughes, "A Study of Temple, Texas During World War II" (Master's, Southwest Texas State University, 1972), 52.
[133] David J. Grettler, "Activity for Body and Mind: The Career of Nora Staael Evert, Physical Therapy Pioneer," *South Dakota History* 47, no. 1 (Spring 2012): 79.
[134] Ibid.
[135] "One Thing Is Sure--Soldier Patients Won't Go Hungry," *Temple Daily Telegram*, November 4, 1942, 12.

[136] Homer G. Olsen, "Food Is Good and Plentiful at McCloskey General Hospital," *The Austin American-Statesman*, March 13, 1944.

[137] Harman, "Professional Services of Dietitians, World War II," 198.

[138] "McCloskey Soldiers Start Move into New Barracks This Week; Library Equipped, Open; Bethea Has Army Anniversary: 92nd's C.O. Now Colonel," *Temple Daily Telegram*, n.d.

[139] James A. Bethea, "Annual Report of McCloskey General Hospital, Temple, Texas For the Calendar Year 1944" (Temple, TX: McCloskey General Hospital, January 1, 1945), 17.

[140] Homer G. Olsen, "Sick Returned to Active Life at McCloskey," *The Austin American-Statesman*, March 8, 1944, 3.

[141] "Hospital's Brig Is in Northeast Corner of Grounds," *Temple Daily Telegram*, November 4, 1942, 1.

[142] James A. Bethea, "Annual Report of McCloskey General Hospital, Temple, Texas For the Calendar Year 1945" (Temple, TX: McCloskey General Hospital, January 1, 1946), 24.

[143] Clifford Joseph Hughes, "A Study of Temple, Texas During World War II" (Master's, San Marcos, TX., Southwest Texas State University, 1972), 52.

[144] Bethea, "Annual Report of McCloskey General Hospital," 29.

[145] James A. Bethea, "Annual Report of McCloskey General Hospital, Temple, Texas For the Calendar Year 1945" (Temple, TX: McCloskey General Hospital, January 1, 1946), 1.

[146] "Civilian Personnel Office Handles All Non-Military Employment at McCloskey," *Temple Daily Telegram*, November 4, 1942, 2.

[147] Augustine Patison, "The Story of Maggie McCloskey" (Olin E. Teague Veterans' Center, n.d.).

[148] "11 Puppies Born to M'Closkey Mascot," N*ewspaper clipping* from Olin E. Teague Veterans' Center Medical Library archives, n.d.

Chapter 5

[149] Rostker, *Providing for the Casualties of War: The American Experience Through World War II, 192*.

[150] Baukhage, "Washington Digest: Today's Battlefield Victims Get Speedy, Effective Care," *The Bartlett Tribune*, December 10, 1943, 2.

[151] Robert S. Gillespie, "Army Hospital Trains," Railway Surgery, 2006, http://railwaysurgery.org/Army.htm, 2.

[152] Lancaster Chapter National Railway Historical Society. Inc., "Trains of Mercy: World War II Hospital Trains," *Lancaster Dispatcher*, September 2013, 3.

[153] Gillespie, 3.

[154] *You're On Your Way.. HOME*, War Department Pamphlet 21–26 (Washington, DC: War Department, 1945), https://archive.org/details/PAM21-26.

[155] United States. Department of the Army, *New Horizons*, War Department Pamphlet 21–17 (Washington, DC: War Department, 1944), http://archive.org/details/PAM21-17.

[156] Homer Olsen, "Teamwork Counts, McCloskey Medical Officer Says, Where Patient Comes First," *The Austin American-Statesman*, March 9, 1944.

[157] Bernard D. Rostker, *Providing for the Casualties of War: The American Experience Through World War II* (Santa Monica, CA.: RAND, c2013), https://www.rand.org/pubs/monographs/MG1164.html, 197.

[158] "3 Troop Carrier Planes Bring 75 Patients to McCloskey," *The Austin American-Statesman*, January 11, 1944.

[159] "375 Soldiers, Ill or Wounded, Moved By Plane," *The Tyler Morning Telegraph*, May 25, 1944, 1.

[160] "Sick and Wounded Sing About Texas As Big Transport Wings Them to McCloskey Hospital," *Corsicana Semi-Weekly Light*, May 26, 1944, 17.

[161] "Malaria Principal Worry of Medics, McCloskey Shows," *The Waco Tribune-Herald*, October 17, 1943, 1.

[162] "Wounded from All Fronts Enter Huge Temple Army Hospital to Leave with Mended Bodies," *The Austin American-Statesman*, July 8, 1943, 2.

[163] "First Baby Born at McCloskey Honored on Birthday Tuesday," *Belton Journal*, November 4, 1943, 3.

[164] Stephen M. Sloan, ed., *Tattooed on My Soul: Texas Veterans Remember World War II* (College Station, Texas: Texas A&M University Press, 2015), 242.

[165] James A. Bethea, "Annual Report of McCloskey General Hospital, Temple, Texas For the Calendar Year 1945" (Temple, TX: McCloskey General Hospital, January 1, 1946), 52.

[166] Hans Pohl and Stephanie Oak, "War & Military Mental Health: The U.S. Psychiatric Response in the 20th Century," *American Journal of Public Health* 97, no. 12 (n.d.): 2135.

[167] Bernard D. Rostker, *Providing for the Casualties of War: The American Experience Through World War II* (Santa Monica, CA.: RAND, c2013), https://www.rand.org/pubs/monographs/MG1164.html, 202.

[168] James A. Bethea, "Annual Report of McCloskey General Hospital, Temple, Texas For the Calendar Year 1944" (Temple, TX: McCloskey General Hospital, January 1, 1945), 41.

[169] Thomas G. E. Wilkes, *Hell's Cauldron* (Atlanta, GA: Stratton-Wilcox, 1953). Wilkes' book is a personal narrative in which he gives" considerable feeling and ill-feeling about his unwarranted and unjust detention" as a psychoneurotic patient at McCloskey and other hospitals.

[170] Bethea, "Annual Report of McCloskey General Hospital, Temple, Texas For the Calendar Year 1945", 73.

[171] James A. Bethea, *Memoirs of James A. Bethea* (San Antonio, TX.: Naylor Co, c1964), 101.

[172] Art Leatherwood, "Camp Swift," in *Handbook of Texas Online*, 2010, https://tshaonline.org/handbook/online/articles/qbc27.

[173] Lyman, Oral History Memoir: Dr. Hannibal (Joe) Jaworski: Interview No. 4, 135.

[174] Bethea, "Annual Report of McCloskey General Hospital, Temple, Texas For the Calendar Year 1945," 100.

[175] Paul J. Dougherty and Marlene DeMaio, "Major General Norman T. Kirk and Amputee Care During World War II," *Clinical Orthopaedics and Related Research*, Symposium: Recent Advances in Amputation Surgery and Rehabilitation, 472, no. 10 (June 6, 2014): 3110, https://doi.org/10.1007/s1199901436796.

[176] Ibid, 3108.

[177] Ibid.

[178] Ibid.

[179] Ibid., 3109.

[180] Ibid., 3110.

[181] Ibid., 3111.

[182] Ibid., 3110.

[183] Emma E. Vogel, Mary S. Lawrence, and Phyllis R. Strobel, "Professional Services of Physical Therapists, World War II," in *Army Medical Specialist Corps*, AMEDD Corps History (Washington, DC: Department of the Army. Office of the Surgeon General; printed by Government Printing Office, 1968), https://history.amedd.army.mil/corps/medical_spec/chaptervii.html, 238-9.

[184] Hal B. Jennings Jr., "Orthopedic Surgery in the Zone of Interior," in *Surgery in World War II*, Medical Department, United States Army (Washington, DC: Office of the Surgeon General, Department of the Army, 1970), 871.

[185] Leonard T. Peterson, "Surgical Consultants in the Zone of Interior. Chapter II: Orthopedic Surgery," in *Activities of Surgical Consultants*, Medical Department, United States Army in World War II (U.S. Army Medical Department, Office of Medical History, 2009), 57.

[186] Army Service Forces, *Meet McGonegal, 1944*, 16 mm, vol. Misc. 956, 2 reels vols., Official Film, War Department (Washington, DC, 1944), https://www.youtube.com/watch?v=FSLj5_HgYlo.

[187] Weldon Hart, "This Man Proves Both Arms Aren't Necessary," *The Austin American-Statesman*, September 13, 1945, sec. Your Capital City, 4.

[188] Jean Begeman, "Lord Halifax's Son, In Witty Speech to Legislature, Praises Texans Fighting in Europe," *The Austin American-Statesman*, March 16, 1945, 8.

[189] "Former GI Keeps Word to Buddies," *The Indiana Gazette*, February 18, 1949, 23.

[190] Begeman, 8.

[191] George Stimpson, "Capital Comment," *The Big Spring Daily Herald*, January 11, 1944, 2.

[192] Emma E. Vogel, Mary S. Lawrence, and Phyllis R. Strobel, "Professional Services of Physical Therapists, World War II," in *Army Medical Specialist Corps*, AMEDD Corps History (Washington, DC: Department of the Army. Office of the Surgeon General; printed by Government Printing Office, 1968), https://history.amedd.army.mil/corps/medical_spec/chaptervii.html, 241.

[193] Weldon Hart, "This Man Proves Both Arms Aren't Necessary," *The Austin American-Statesman*, September 13, 1945, sec. Your Capital City, 4.

[194] "Fort Sam Houston Wins Softball Title," *The Shreveport Journal*, August 29, 1944, 9.

[195] "Maimed Veterans Invent Wheel-Chair Ball Game," *The New York Times*, October 25, 1945, 23.

[196] "No Limbs Needed In This Baseball Loop," *El Paso Times*, October 28, 1945, 16.

[197] James A. Bethea, "Annual Report of McCloskey General Hospital, Temple, Texas For the Calendar Year 1945" (Temple, TX: McCloskey General Hospital, January 1, 1946), 13.

[198] "Convalescing GIs Building Their Own Christmas At Army Hospital," *Lubbock Avalanche-Journal*, December 9, 1945.

[199] "Texas Farm News," *Belton Journal*, May 20, 1943, 10.

[200] "McCloskey Soldier-Patients Appointed Hospital Guides," *The Austin American-Statesman*, May 21, 1944, 5.

[201] *Music in Reconditioning in ASF Convalescent and General Hospitals*. Technical Bulletin, TB Med 187. Washington, DC: War Department, 1945, 1.

[202] James A. Bethea, "Annual Report of McCloskey General Hospital, Temple, Texas For the Calendar Year 1944" (Temple, TX: McCloskey General Hospital, January 1, 1945), 14.

[203] Bethea and Ellis, 103.

[204] Sloan, *Tattooed on My Soul*, 244.

[205] Ibid., 242.

[206] Daniel Lyman, Oral History Memoir: Dr. Hannibal (Joe) Jaworski: Interview No. 4, March 9, 1990, Baylor University Institute for Oral History, 132.

[207] Sloan, *Tattooed on My Soul*, 243.

[208] Ibid., 244.

[209] Daniel Lyman, Oral History Memoir: Dr. Hannibal (Joe) Jaworski: Interview No. 4, March 9, 1990, Baylor University Institute for Oral History, 127.

[210] "3 Day Conference M'Closkey Hospital," *Corsicana Daily Sun*, January 26, 1945, 3.

[211] "Major Gen. Kirk Visits McCloskey," *The Belton Journal and Bell County Democrat*, October 11, 1945, 7.

[212] Jennings, "Orthopedic Surgery in the Zone of Interior", 482.

[213] Ibid., 906.

[214] "Army Seeks Better Limbs For Wounded," *Waxahachie Daily Light*, March 19, 1946, 8.

[215] Walter R. Humphrey, "Wounded Don't Want Stares; Just A Chance to Get Along," *The Palm Beach Post*, June 10, 1945, 11.

Chapter 7

[216] Daniel Lyman, Oral History Memoir: Dr. Hannibal (Joe) Jaworski: Interview No. 4, March 9, 1990, Baylor University Institute for Oral History, 129.

[217] Sloan, *Tattooed on My Soul*, 244.

[218] Patricia K. Benoit, "Backroads: Penicillin Was Lifesaver to Soldiers During World War II," *Temple Daily Telegram*, May 27, 2019, 3A.

[219] "Malaria Principal Worry of Medics, McCloskey Shows," *The Waco Tribune-Herald*, October 17, 1943, 6.

[220] James A. Bethea, "Annual Report of McCloskey General Hospital, Temple, Texas For the Calendar Year 1944" (Temple, TX: McCloskey General Hospital, January 1, 1945), 64.

[221] "Penicillin Soon to Be Available in Ample Quantity," *The Morning Call*, December 14, 1943.

[222] Baukhage, 2."

[223] "Developments in Military Medicine During the Administration of Major General Norman T. Kirk," *Bulletin of the U.S. Army Medical Department* 7 (1947): 594–646. The greatest quantitative use of penicillin was in the treatment of gonorrhea and syphilis.

[224] Clifford Joseph Hughes, "A Study of Temple, Texas During World War II" (Master's, Southwest Texas State University, 1972), 53.

[225] "How Army Dentists Broke Nazi's Glass Eye Monopoly: Wounded Soldiers Faced Black Patches Until They Developed New Plastics," *The Milwaukee Journal*, April 26, 1945, 47.

[226] "Hearst Charge of Neglected Soldier Branded as False," *The Pittsburgh Press*, March 5, 1944, 2.

[227] Homer G. Olsen, "Former Hearst Writer Upholds Officers of Hospital Staff," *The Pittsburgh Press*, March 5, 1944.

[228] Dick Pearce, "Army Gives Refund to Disabled McCloud Vet," *San Francisco Examiner*, February 19, 1944, 7.

[229] William McCullam, "Hands Gone, Blind, Deaf, Boy Left to Shift for Himself by Army," *San Francisco Examiner*, January 25, 1944, 16.

[230] "First Case." *Time Magazine*, July 23, 1945, 77.

[231] *McCloskey General Hospital, Temple, Texas* (S.l.: United States Army, 194?), 12.

[232] Gerald L. Burke, "The Corrosion of Metals in Tissues; and An Introduction to Tantalum," *Canadian Medical Association Journal* 43, no. 2 (August 1940): 128.

[233] "New Magic Metal Working Miracles for War Wounded," *Lubbock Morning Avalanche*, February 8, 1944. 2.

[234] Bethea, "Annual Report of McCloskey General Hospital, Temple, Texas For the Calendar Year 1944," 99.

[235] Janice S. Todd, Jason P. Shurley, and Terry C. Todd, "Thomas L. DeLorme and the Science of Progressive Resistance Exercise," *The Journal of Strength & Conditioning Research* 26, no. 11 (November 2012): 2913–2923, https://doi.org/10.1519/JSC.0b013e31825adcb4.

[236] Bernard D. Rostker, *Providing for the Casualties of War: The American Experience Through World War II* (Santa Monica, CA.: RAND, c2013), https://www.rand.org/pubs/monographs/MG1164.html, 190.

[237] David Dietz, "Army Doctors," *The Pittsburgh Press*, April 22, 1944, sec. Science Today.

[238] Robert Davies, *Baldwin of the Times: Hanson W. Baldwin, a Military Journalist's Life, 1903-1991* (New York, NY.: Naval Institute Press, 2013), 125.

[239] "Floodlighted Ball Field in Temple Available for Central Texas Towns," *The Belton Journal and Bell County Democrat*, September 23, 1948, 2.

[240] "McCloskey Patients Get $206.75 From Local Benefit Dance," *West News*, December 8, 1944, 1.

[241] "Salerno Veterans Guests of Nation," *Nebraska State Journal*, December 24, 1943, 2.

[242] "Soldiers in Texas Army Hospitals Have Good Christmas With Home Only In Their Dreams," *The Austin American-Statesman*, December 26, 1943, 1.

[243] "Catholic Women Here Send Largest Cookie Jar to McCloskey," *The Cameron Herald*, March 1, 1945, 5.

[244] "To Boys at McCloskey," *The Austin American-Statesman*, December 23, 1943, sec. Town Talk, 1, 17.

[245] "Flowers for the Road Back: Texas Rotarians Provide a Veterans Hospital with a Modern Greenhouse," *The Rotarian*, March 1947, 43.

[246] John Strege, *When War Played Through: Golf During World War II*, Reprint edition (Gotham Books, 2006), 283.

[247] "Slammin' Snead Exhibits Shots for McCloskey," *Abilene Reporter-News*, September 11, 1945, 8.

[248] "VA Hospital in Temple to Stage State Golf Meet," *Waco News-Tribune*, August 10, 1946, 11.

[249] Victor E. Schulze, Jr., *U.S. Army McCloskey General Hospital: 1942-1946, Temple, Texas* ([United States]: s.n, 1993?), 36.

[250] "James E. Ferguson, Former Texas Governor, Dies at Austin Home," *Borger Daily Herald*, September 22, 1944, 1.

[251] "Landscape Project Brings Contributions," *The Austin American-Statesman*, November 12, 1944, 3.

[252] "A.A.U.W. Hears of Red Cross Work in County," *Belton Journal and Bell County Democrat*, November 12, 1942, 1.

[253] "Belton Red Cross Lagging in Making Surgical Dressings," *The Belton Journal and Bell County Democrat*, February 25, 1943, 1.

[254] "Mary Lela Engvall," *The Austin American-Statesman*, October 8, 1995, sec. Obituaries, 28.

[255] "Gray Ladies Ranks Thinned by Season," *The Belton Journal and Bell County Democrat*, July 26, 1945, 1. "Grey Ladies" is an alternate spelling found in some sources.

[256] James A. Bethea, "Annual Report of McCloskey General Hospital, Temple, Texas For the Calendar Year 1945" (Temple, TX: McCloskey General Hospital, January 1, 1946), 30.

[257] "Red Cross Still Has Many Calls For Its Services: Post-War Needs Keeps Bell County Chapter Very Busy," *The Belton Journal and Bell County Democrat*, December 19, 1946, 7.

[258] Raymond Brooks, "Former Head of 36th Sees His Wounded," *The Austin American-Statesman*, August 17, 1944, 2.

[259] "Johnson Urges Continued Work On Home Front," *The Austin American-Statesman*, December 23, 1943, 2.

[260] Helen Selsdon, "Helen Keller and the American Foundation for the Blind's Commitment to Veterans Who Have Lost Their Sight," *American Foundation for the Blind* (blog), November 10, 2014, https://www.afb.org/blog/entry/helen-keller-and-american-foundation-blinds-commitment-veterans.

[261] James A. Bethea, "Letter from James A. Bethea, Commanding General, McCloskey General Hospital, Temple, TX. to Helen Keller, New York, NY.," Typewritten, November

27, 1944, American Foundation for the Blind, https://bit.ly/3aLgN2z

[262] "Bobby Byrne's Skyliners Will Play at McCloskey," *The Austin American-Statesman*, June 26, 1944, 3.

[263] Thomas F. Sliger, "48 Hours in Paradise," *The Rotarian*, January 1946.

[264] "Texas Inland Fishing Outlook Good as Summer Moves In," *Abilene Reporter-News*, May 25, 1945, 8.

[265] "They Still Know How to Shoot," *The Austin American-Statesman*, January 3, 1945, 7.

[266] "Officials at McCloskey Cancel Minstrel Show," *Taylor Daily Press*, April 8, 1945, 4.

[267] John Vernon, "Jim Crow, Meet Lieutenant Robinson: A 1944 Court-Martial," *Prologue Magazine*, Spring 2008, https://www.archives.gov/publications/prologue/2008/spring/robinson.html.

[268] "McCloskey Patient Marries at USO," *Belton Journal and Bell County Democrat*, August 2, 1945, 5. They remained married and are buried together in Hampton City, VA.

[269] "McCloskey Reconditions Vets for Civilian Life," *Denton Record-Chronicle*, July 13, 1945, sec. Texas Today, 4.

[270] "Kindness, Happiness, Efficiency, Principles Underlying Treatment of Veterans at McCloskey General," *The Eagle*, July 19, 1945, 3. Edwards was known as the human booby trap because Germans wired him with booby traps when he was helpless with wounds.

[271] Fred D. Thompson, "Wounded War Heroes From McCloskey To Help Austin Launch Bond Campaign," *The Austin American-Statesman*, January 11, 1944, 1.

[272] "McCloskey Vets Push 5th Loan," *The Austin American-Statesman*, August 11, 1944, 6.

[273] Clifford Joseph Hughes, "A Study of Temple, Texas During World War II" (Master's, Southwest Texas State University, 1972), 55.

[274] James A. Bethea, "Annual Report of McCloskey General Hospital, Temple, Texas For the Calendar Year 1945" (Temple, TX: McCloskey General Hospital, January 1, 1946), 6.

[275] "Lou Gehrig Trophy Auctioned Off at War Bond Fight," *The Big Spring Daily Herald*, June 21, 1944. 9.

[276] Raymond Brooks, "Cheery Spirit Dominant In Army Hospital," *The Austin American-Statesman*, August 18, 1944, sec. Texas Topics, 4.

[277] "The Texan's Share In Winning World War 2," *The Denison Press*, September 8, 1944, 3.

Chapter 8

David Dietz, "Army Doctors," *The Pittsburgh Press*, April 22, 1944, sec. Science Today.

"Floodlighted Ball Field in Temple Available for Central Texas Towns," *The Belton Journal and Bell County Democrat*, September 23, 1948, 2.

"McCloskey Patients Get $206.75 From Local Benefit Dance," *West News*, December 8, 1944, 1.

"Salerno Veterans Guests of Nation," *Nebraska State Journal*, December 24, 1943, 2.

"Soldiers in Texas Army Hospitals Have Good Christmas With Home Only in Their Dreams," *The Austin American-Statesman*, December 26, 1943, 1.

"Catholic Women Here Send Largest Cookie Jar to McCloskey," *The Cameron Herald*, March 1, 1945, 5.

"To Boys at McCloskey," *The Austin American-Statesman*, December 23, 1943, sec. Town Talk, 1, 17.

"Flowers for the Road Back: Texas Rotarians Provide a Veterans Hospital with a Modern Greenhouse," *The Rotarian*, March 1947, 43.

John Strege, *When War Played Through: Golf During World War II*, Reprint edition (Gotham Books, 2006), 283.

"Slammin' Snead Exhibits Shots for McCloskey," *Abilene Reporter-News*, September 11, 1945, 8.

"VA Hospital in Temple to Stage State Golf Meet," *Waco News-Tribune*, August 10, 1946, 11.

Victor E. Schulze, Jr., *U.S. Army McCloskey General Hospital: 1942-1946, Temple, Texas* ([United States]: s.n, 1993?), 36.

"James E. Ferguson, Former Texas Governor, Dies at Austin Home," *Borger Daily Herald*, September 22, 1944, 1.

"Landscape Project Brings Contributions," *The Austin American-Statesman*, November 12, 1944, 3.

"A.A.U.W. Hears of Red Cross Work in County," *The Belton Journal and Bell County Democrat*, November 12, 1942, 1.

"Belton Red Cross Lagging in Making Surgical Dressings," *The Belton Journal and Bell County Democrat,* February 25, 1943, 1.

"Mary Lela Engvall," *The Austin American-Statesman*, October 8, 1995, sec. Obituaries, 28.

"Gray Ladies Ranks Thinned by Season," *The Belton Journal and Bell County Democrat*, July 26, 1945, 1. "Grey Ladies" is an alternate spelling found in some sources.

James A. Bethea, "Annual Report of McCloskey General Hospital, Temple, Texas For the Calendar Year 1945" (Temple, TX: McCloskey General Hospital, January 1, 1946), 30.

"Red Cross Still Has Many Calls for Its Services: Post-War Needs Keeps Bell County Chapter Very Busy," *The Belton Journal and Bell County Democrat*, December 19, 1946, 7.

Chapter 9

Raymond Brooks, "Former Head of 36th Sees His Wounded," *The Austin American-Statesman*, August 17, 1944, 2.

"Johnson Urges Continued Work on Home Front," *The Austin American-Statesman,* December 23, 1943, 2.

Helen Selsdon, "Helen Keller and the American Foundation for the Blind's Commitment to Veterans Who Have Lost Their Sight," American Foundation for the Blind (blog), November 10, 2014, https://www.afb.org/blog/entry/helen-keller-and-american-foundation-blinds-commitment-veterans.

James A. Bethea, "Letter from James A. Bethea, Commanding General, McCloskey General Hospital, Temple, TX. to Helen Keller, New York, NY.," Typewritten, November 27, 1944, American Foundation for the Blind, https://bit.ly/3aLgN2z

"Bobby Byrne's Skyliners Will Play at McCloskey," *The Austin American-Statesman*, June 26, 1944, 3.

Thomas F. Sliger, "48 Hours in Paradise," *The Rotarian*, January 1946.

"Texas Inland Fishing Outlook Good as Summer Moves In," *Abilene Reporter-News*, May 25, 1945, 8.

"They Still Know How to Shoot," *The Austin American-Statesman*, January 3, 1945, 7.

"Officials at McCloskey Cancel Minstrel Show," *Taylor Daily Press*, April 8, 1945, 4.

John Vernon, "Jim Crow, Meet Lieutenant Robinson: A 1944 Court-Martial," *Prologue Magazine*, Spring 2008, https://www.archives.gov/publications/prologue/2008/spring/robinson.html.

"McCloskey Patient Marries at USO," *The Belton Journal and Bell County Democrat*, August 2, 1945, 5. They remained married and are buried together in Hampton City, VA.

"McCloskey Reconditions Vets for Civilian Life," *Denton Record-Chronicle,* July 13, 1945, sec. Texas Today, 4.

"Kindness, Happiness, Efficiency, Principles Underlying Treatment of Veterans at McCloskey General," *The Eagle*, July 19, 1945, 3. Edwards was known as the human booby trap because Germans wired him with booby traps when he was helpless with wounds.

Fred D. Thompson, "Wounded War Heroes from McCloskey To Help Austin Launch Bond Campaign," *The Austin American-Statesman*, January 11, 1944, 1.

"McCloskey Vets Push 5th Loan," *The Austin American-Statesman,* August 11, 1944, 6.

Clifford Joseph Hughes, "A Study of Temple, Texas During World War II" (Master's, Southwest Texas State University, 1972), 55.

James A. Bethea, "Annual Report of McCloskey General Hospital, Temple, Texas For the Calendar Year 1945" (Temple, TX: McCloskey General Hospital, January 1, 1946), 6.

"Lou Gehrig Trophy Auctioned Off at War Bond Fight," *The Big Spring Daily Herald*, June 21, 1944. 9.

Raymond Brooks, "Cheery Spirit Dominant in Army Hospital," *The Austin American-Statesman*, August 18, 1944, sec. Texas Topics, 4.

"The Texan's Share in Winning World War 2," *The Denison Press*, September 8, 1944, 3.

Chapter 10

[278] Kurt Gregory, "The German World War Two Prisoner and His Experience in the United States" (Master's, California State University, 2001), 17.

[279] Walker, Richard Paul, "Prisoners of War in Texas During World War II" (Dissertation, North Texas State University, 1980), 99. General Bethea stated in his *Annual Report* of 1945 that "Among other items, a new Prisoner of War Camp was constructed."

[280] Richard P. Walker, *The Lone Star and the Swastika: Prisoners of War in Texas* (Austin, TX: Eakin Press, c2001), 45.

[281] Walker, Richard Paul, "Prisoners of War in Texas During World War II," 99.

[282] Ibid.

[283] Carol Mouche, "Area Residents Recall Temple's Prisoner-of-War Camp," *Temple Daily Telegram*, May 5, 1985.

[284] "Fatal Beating of War Prisoner at Hearne Eyed," *The Austin American-Statesman*, January 14, 1944, 15..

[285] Clay Coppedge, "Temple Camp Housed German, Italian Prisoners," *Temple Daily Telegram*, May 20, 2007.

[286] Clay Coppedge, "Lanky and the POWs," *Texas Escapes Online Magazine*, November 8, 2006, sec. Letters from Central Texas, http://www.texasescapes.com/ClayCoppedge/Lanky-and-the-POWs.htm.

[287] William C. Barnard, "Every Prisoner of War Escaping From Camps Recaptured," *Corsicana Daily Sun*, May 1, 1944, 1.

[288] Jenny Ashcraft, "WWII POW Camps in the United States," *Fold3 Blog* (blog), August 8, 2019, https://blog.fold3.com/wwii-pow-camps-in-the-united-states/.

[289] Gregory, "The German World War Two Prisoner and His Experience in the United States", 29.

[290] William C. Barnard, "Prisoners of War in Texas Rapidly Being Repatriated," *The Denton Record-Chronicle*, January 1, 1946.

Chapter 11

[291] James A. Bethea, *Memoirs of James A. Bethea* (San Antonio, TX.: Naylor Co, c1964), 103-104.

[292] "Battle-Scarred Heroes of Fighting 36th Tell of Grim Salerno Landing," *Paris News*, November 15, 1943, 1.

[293] "High-Ranking Officers With Fifth Army In Italy Arrive At McCloskey Hospital; Tell of Terrible Battles," *The Tyler Morning Telegraph*, April 25, 1944, 5.

[294] "Wife Already Knew Soldier Had Lost Leg," *The Austin American-Statesman*, April 10, 1944, 2.

[295] "Gordon P. Roman in Rome Invasion," *The Longview News Journal*, August 4, 1944, 5.

[296] Walter R. Humphrey, "First Invasion Casualties Normandy Beaches Reach Hospital in Temple Tuesday," *Corsicana Daily Sun*, July 11, 1944, 12.

[297] "Men From Nazi Camps Arrive at McCloskey," *Abilene Reporter-News*, March 5, 1945, 16.

[298] "Skin and Bones Pictures Show True Prison Situation," *The Belton Journal and Bell County Democrat*, March 29, 1945, 2.

[299] "Returnee From Jap Prison Is Head Dietitian at McCloskey," *The Belton Journal and Bell County Democrat*, October 4, 1945, 7.

[300] "Lost Battalion Texans at Temple," *The Monitor*, October 24, 1945, 5.

[301] "The Facts About John Lindsey's Baseball Wound," *The Big Spring Daily Herald*, March 6, 1945, 13.

[302] "Wounded From All Fronts Enter Huge Temple Army Hospital To Leave With Mended Bodies," *The Austin American-Statesman*, July 8, 1943, 2.

[303] "Pvt. WAAC Dog Veteran of Attu Fight At Hospital Here," *Temple Daily Telegram*, June 16, 1943, 1.

[304] "McCloskey Hospital Has Patients from Every Battlefront of This War," *El Paso Times*, May 21, 1944. 13.

[305] "Broken in Body But Not in Spirit," *St. Cloud Times*, September 25, 1945.

[306] "Hero Tells Why Divorce Suit Filed," *The Austin American-Statesman*, August 1, 1945, 5.

Chapter 12

[307] "Request for Use Of McCloskey By V A Awaits Action," *The Austin American-Statesman*, March 19, 1946, sec. Editorials, 4.

[308] James A. Bethea, "Annual Report of McCloskey General Hospital, Temple, Texas For the Calendar Year 1945" (Temple, TX: McCloskey General Hospital, January 1, 1946), 2.

[309] James A. Bethea, *Memoirs of James A. Bethea* (San Antonio, TX.: Naylor Co, c1964), 106-7.

[310] "McCloskey Hospital Put Back in Service," *The Austin American-Statesman*, April 4, 1946, 4.

[311] Victor E. Schulze, Jr., *U.S. Army McCloskey General Hospital, 1942-1946, Temple, Texas* ([United States]: s.n., 1993?), 42.

[312] "Gen. Bradley, V A Head, Makes Inspection Trip," *The Richland Beacon News*, April 27, 1946, 6.

[313] Harry S. Truman, "Rear Platform and Other Informal Remarks in Texas | Harry S. Truman," Truman Library, September 27, 1948, https://www.trumanlibrary.gov/library/public-papers/212/rear-platform-and-other-informal-remarks-texas.

[314] Tex Easley, "VA Hospital Needs to Be Checked," *The Austin American-Statesman*, December 1, 1948, 10.

[315] "McCloskey Needs Nurses to Expand Services to Vets," *The Waco News-Tribune*, September 28, 1946, 7.

[316] Dan A. Sebek, "Veterans Administration Memorandum to Chief, Voluntary Service Re: Historical Information," November 9, 1981.

[317] "Shivers, Civic Leaders Battle Over Hospital," *El Paso Times*, October 10, 1952, 6.

[318] Ibid.

[319] "Shivers, Civic Leaders Battle Over Hospital," *El Paso Times*, October 10, 1952, 6.

[320] "Dispute Over Moving TB Patients Grows; Poage's Remark Hit," *Brownwood Bulletin*, October 17, 1952, 3.

[321] W. R. Poage, "Letter from W. R. Poage to Hon. R. C. Tompkins," October 17, 1952, Olin E. Teague Veterans' Administration Center Medical Library Archives, 2.

[322] "Temple Fight To End With VA Decision," *The Waco News-Tribune*, October 11, 1952, 1.

[323] Ernest L. Wilkinson, "The United States Court of Claims: Where Uncle Sam Is Always the Defendant," *American Bar Association Journal* 36 (February 1950), 155.

[324] American Const. Co. v. United States, 123 Ct. Cl. 408 (United States Court of Claims 1952), 4.

[325] Ibid., 16.

[326] Alec Philmore Pearson Jr., "Olin E. Teague and the Veterans' Administration" (Texas A&M University, 1977), 235.

[327] Ibid., 245.

[328] "McCloskey VA Center Cited for Efficiency," *The Waco Tribune-Herald*, October 2, 1960, 22A.

[329] "Temple, Tex. Land Conveyance," Pub. L. No. 90–197, 81 STAT. U.S. Code 582 (1967).

[330] Melanie Watkins, "Teague, Olin Earl [Tiger]," in *Handbook of Texas Online* (Texas State Historical Association, n.d.), accessed October 16, 2019.

[331] Pearson, "Olin E. Teague and the Veterans' Administration," 11.

[332] "Solon Proposes To Name McCloskey For 36th Division," *Waco News-Tribune*, March 21, 1947, 11.

[333] Clifford Joseph Hughes, "A Study of Temple, Texas During World War II" (Master's, Southwest Texas State University, 1972), 88.

Bibliography

Blogs

Ashcraft, Jenny. "WWII POW Camps in the United States."
Fold3 Blog (blog), August 8, 2019.
https://blog.fold3.com/wwii-pow-camps-in-the-united-
states/.

Batens, Alain S., and Ben C. Major. "WW2 Military Hospitals.
Zone of Interior (United States)." *WW2 US Medical
Research Centre* (blog). Accessed January 25, 2019.
https://www.med-dept.com/articles/ww2-military-
hospitals-zone-of-interior/.

WW2 US Medical Research Centre. "Brief Overview of the
Medical Department." Accessed February 21, 2019.
https://www.med-dept.com/articles/brief-overview-of-
the-medical-department/.

PTTransforms Staff. "Remembering the Reconstruction Aides."
#PTTransforms (blog), March 9, 2018.
http://www.apta.org/Blogs/PTTransforms/2018/3/8/Re
constructionAides/.

Selsdon, Helen. "'An Incalculable Debt We Owe You': Helen
Keller on Veterans Day." *American Foundation for the
Blind* (blog), November 10, 2015.
https://www.afb.org/blog/afb-blog/an-incalculable-
debt-we-owe-you-helen-keller-on-veterans-day/12.

———. "Helen Keller and the American Foundation for the
Blind's Commitment to Veterans Who Have Lost Their
Sight." *American Foundation for the Blind* (blog),
November 10, 2014.
https://www.afb.org/blog/entry/helen-keller-and-
american-foundation-blinds-commitment-veterans.

Sparrow, Paul M. "The 'Four Freedoms' Speech Remastered."
*Forward with Roosevelt: The Blog of the Franklin D.
Roosevelt Presidential Library and Museum* (blog),
January 6, 2016.
https://fdr.blogs.archives.gov/2016/01/06/four_freedo

ms/.

Texas Historical Commission. "Texas in World War II." *Real Places Telling Real Stories* (blog), 2019. https://www.thc.texas.gov/preserve/projects-and-programs/military-sites/texas-world-war-ii.

Book Chapters

Brosin, Henry W. "Zone of Interior. Pt. 3. Military Psychiatry in Practice. Chapter XI: General Hospitals." In *Neuropsychiatry in World War II*, Vol. 1, n.d. https://history.amedd.army.mil/booksdocs/wwii/Neuro psychiatryinWWIIVol1/chapter11.htm.

Coates, John Boyd, and Elizabeth M. McFetridge. "Blood Program in World War II." In *Medical Department, United States Army*, 968. Washington, DC: Department of the Army. Office of the Surgeon General; printed by Government Printing Office, 1964.

"Defense Measures of the United States 1940." In *Peace and War: United States Foreign Policy, 1931-1941*. United States. Department of State Publication 1983. Washington, DC: Government Printing Office, 1943. https://www.mtholyoke.edu/acad/intrel/WorldWar2/d efense.htm.

Duryea, E. A. "A General's Journey-Norman T. Kirk." In *The Surgeons General of the U.S. Army and Their Predecessors: Norman Thomas Kirk*. Washington, DC: Department of the Army. Office of the Surgeon General; printed by Government Printing Office, n.d. https://history.amedd.army.mil/surgeongenerals/N_Kir k3.html.

Harman, Thelma A. "Professional Services of Dietitians, World War II." In *Army Medical Specialist Corps*. AMEDD Corps History. Washington, DC: Department of the Army. Office of the Surgeon General; printed by Government Printing Office, 1968. https://history.amedd.army.mil/corps/medical_spec/ch

aptervii.html.

Jennings, Hal B., Jr. "Orthopedic Surgery in the Zone of
Interior." In *Surgery in World War II*. Medical
Department, United States Army. Washington, DC:
Office of the Surgeon General, Department of Army,
1970.

"Norman Thomas Kirk." In *The Surgeons General of the U.S.
Army and Their Predecessors:* Washington, DC:
Department of the Army. Office of the Surgeon
General; printed by Government Printing Office, n.d.
https://history.amedd.army.mil/surgeongenerals/N_Kir
k2.html.

Peterson, Leonard T. "Surgical Consultants in the Zone of
Interior. Chapter II: Orthopedic Surgery." In *Activities of
Surgical Consultants*. Medical Department, United
States Army in World War II. U.S. Army Medical
Department, Office of Medical History, 2009.

Vogel, Emma E., Mary S. Lawrence, and Phyllis R. Strobel.
"Professional Services of Physical Therapists, World
War II." In *Army Medical Specialist Corps*. AMEDD Corps
History. Washington, DC: Department of the Army.
Office of the Surgeon General; printed by Government
Printing Office, 1968.
https://history.amedd.army.mil/corps/medical_spec/ch
apterviii.html.

Vogel, Emma E., Katherine E. Manchester, Helen B. Gearin, and
Wilma L. West. "Training in World War II." In *Army
Medical Specialist Corps*. AMEDD Corps History.
Washington, DC: Department of the Army. Office of the
Surgeon General; printed by Government Printing
Office, 1968.
https://history.amedd.army.mil/corps/medical_spec/ch
aptervi.html.

Books

Ambrose, Stephen E. *D-Day, June 6, 1944: The Climactic Battle of World War II*. New York: Simon & Schuster, 1994.

Barrett, Christina M. *Dreeben-Irimia's Introduction to Physical Therapist Practice for Physical Therapist Assistants*. 3rd ed. Burlington, MA: Jones and Bartlett, 2016.

Beebe, Gilbert W., and Michael E. DeBakey. *Battle Casualties, Incidence, Mortality, and Logistic Considerations*, Springfield, IL: Charles C. Thomas, 1952. https://babel.hathitrust.org/cgi/pt?id=inu.32000014231783;view=1up;seq=1.

Bellafaire, Judith A. *The Army Nurse Corps: A Commemoration of World War II Service*. Center of Military History Publication, CMH Pub 72-14. U.S. Army Center of Military History, 2003. https://history.army.mil/books/wwii/72-14/72-14.HTM.

Bethea, James A. *Memoirs of James A. Bethea*. San Antonio, Tex: Naylor Co, 1964.

Davies, Robert. *Baldwin of the Times: Hanson W. Baldwin, a Military Journalist's Life, 1903-1991*. New York, NY.: Naval Institute Press, 2013.

Dillingham, Timothy R., and Praxedes V. Belandres. *Rehabilitation of the Injured Combatant*. Textbook of Military Medicine, Part IV, Surgical Combat Casualty Care. Washington, DC: Office of the Surgeon General at TMM Publications, Borden Institute, Walter Reed Army Medical Center, 1998.

Educational Reconditioning. Technical Manual, TM 8-290. Washington, DC: War Department, 1944.

Fath, Shudde Bess Bryson, and Betsy Fath Hiller. *The Greatest Generation as Reported in the Weekly Bastrop Adviser During World War II*. S.l.: Xlibris Corporation, c2011.

Faulk, Odie B., and Laura E. Faulk, *Frank W. Mayborn: A Man Who Made a Difference*. Belton, TX: University of Mary Hardin-Baylor, 1989.

Federal Security Agency. Public Health Service. *The United States Cadet Nurse Corps [1943-1948] and Other Federal Nurse Training Programs*. PHS Publication No. 38. Washington, DC: Government Printing Office, 1950.

http://archive.org/details/CadetNurseCorps1943-1948.

Helpful Hints to Those Who Have Lost Limbs. War Department
Pamphlet, No. 8-7. Washington, DC: War Department,
1944.
https://collections.nlm.nih.gov/catalog/nlm:nlmuid-
36210370R-bk.

Kelsey, Michael. *Temple*. Images of America. Charleston, S.C.:
Arcadia Publishing, 2010.

King, John E., and Raymond G. Hynson. *Highlights in the History
of U.S. Army Dentistry*. Falls Church, VA: U.S. Army,
Office of the Surgeon General, 2007.

Lewis, George G., and John Mewha. *History of Prisoner of War
Utilization by The United States Army 1776-1945*. DA
Pamphlet 20–213. Washington, DC: Department of the
Army, 1955.

Matloff, Maurice, and Edwin M. Snell. *Strategic Planning for
Coalition Warfare 1941-1942*. Washington, DC: United
States Army. Center of Military History, 1990.
https://history.army.mil/books/wwii/SP1941-
42/index.htm#Contents.

McCloskey General Hospital, Temple, Texas [Christmas Menu].
S.l.: United States Army, 194AD.

Mullins, William S., and Robert J. Parks. *Medical Training in
World War II*. Medical Department, United States Army.
Washington, DC: U.S. Army, Office of the Surgeon
General, 1974.

*Music in Reconditioning in ASF Convalescent and General
Hospitals*. Technical Bulletin, TB Med 187. Washington,
DC: War Department, 1945.

Office of War Information. *Information Program for the United
States Cadet Nurse Corps*. Washington, DC:
Government Printing Office, 1943.

Peace and War, United States Foreign Policy, 1931-1941.
United States. Department of State Publication 1983.
Washington, DC: Government Printing Office, 1943.
https://hdl.handle.net/2027/mdp.39015023272209.

Rodeman, Charlotte R. *Neuropsychiatry in World War II*. *Pt. IV:*

Supporting Services and Personnel. U.S. Army Medical Department. Office of Medical History., 2009. https://history.amedd.army.mil/booksdocs/wwii/Neuro psychiatryinWWIIVoII/DEFAULT.htm.

Rostker, Bernard D. *Providing for the Casualties of War: The American Experience Through World War II*. Santa Monica, CA.: RAND, c2013. https://www.rand.org/pubs/monographs/MG1164.htm l.

Schulze, Jr., Victor E. *U.S. Army McCloskey General Hospital, 1942-1946, Temple, Texas*. [United States]: s.n., 1993?

Sloan, Stephen M., ed. *Tattooed on My Soul: Texas Veterans Remember World War II*. College Station, TX.: Texas A&M University Press, 2015.

Small Army Libraries. War Department Technical Manual, TM 28-305. Washington, DC: Government Printing Office, 1944.

Smith, Clarence McKittrick. *The Medical Department: Hospitalization and Evacuation, Zone of Interior*. United States Army in World War II. Washington: Office of the Chief of Military History, Dept. of the Army, 1956.

Strege, John. *When War Played Through: Golf During World War II*. Reprint edition. Gotham Books, 2006.

The Templar: Yearbook of Temple Junior College, 1939/1940. Temple, TX: Temple Junior College, 1940. https://texashistory.unt.edu/ark:/67531/metapth9790 01/: accessed December 16, 2019), University of North Texas Libraries, The Portal to Texas History, https://texashistory.unt.edu.

United States Census Bureau. *1950 Census of Population: Volume 1. Number of Inhabitants. Texas*. Washington, DC: Government Printing Office, n.d. https.//www2.census.gov/library/publications/decenni al/1950/population-volume-1/vol-01-46.pdf.

United States. Department of the Army. *New Horizons*. War Department Pamphlet 21–17. Washington, DC: War Department, 1944. http://archive.org/details/PAM21-

17.

Walker, Richard P. *The Lone Star and the Swastika: Prisoners of War in Texas*. Austin, TX: Eakin Press, c2001.

Wilkes, Thomas G. E. *Hell's Cauldron*. Atlanta, GA: Stratton-Wilcox, 1953.

You're on Your Way... HOME. War Department Pamphlet 21–26. Washington, DC: War Department, 1945. https://archive.org/details/PAM21-26.

Encyclopedia Articles

Cohen, Judith S. "Geren, Preston Murdoch, Sr." In *Handbook of Texas Online*. Texas State Historical Association, 2010. https://tshaonline.org/handbook/online/articles/fge17.

———. "Pelich, Joseph Roman." In *Handbook of Texas Online*. Texas State Historical Association, June 15, 2010. http://www.tshaonline.org/handbook/online/articles/fpepv.

Leatherwood, Art. "Camp Swift." In *Handbook of Texas Online*. Texas State Historical Association, 2010. https://tshaonline.org/handbook/online/articles/qbc27.

Smyrl, Vivian Elizabeth. "Temple, Texas." In *Handbook of Texas Online*. Texas State Historical Association, June 15, 2010. https://tshaonline.org/handbook/online/articles/hdt01.

Watkins, Melanie. "Teague, Olin Earl [Tiger]." In *Handbook of Texas Online*. Texas State Historical Association, n.d. Accessed October 16, 2019.

Interviews

Lyman, Daniel. Oral History Memoir: Dr. Hannibal (Joe) Jaworski: Interview No. 3, March 2, 1990. Baylor University Institute for Oral History.

———. Oral History Memoir: Dr. Hannibal (Joe) Jaworski: Interview No. 4, March 9, 1990. Baylor University

Institute for Oral History.

Journal Articles

"Army Develops Superior Artificial Eyes." *Bulletin of the U.S. Army Medical Department*, no. No. 86 (March 1945): 12.

Arnaud, Celia Henry. "Penicillin." *Chemical & Engineering News* 83, no. 25 (June 20, 2005). https://cen.acs.org/content/cen/articles/83/i25/Penicill in.html.

Burke, Gerald L. "The Corrosion of Metals in Tissues; and An Introduction to Tantalum." *Canadian Medical Association Journal* 43, no. 2 (August 1940): 125–28.

Carpentier, Gaetan. "Casualty of History: A WWII Prisoner of War Grave at the San Antonio National Cemetery." *Intersect: Perspectives in Texas Public History* 2, no. 1 (2015): 5–12.

"Developments in Military Medicine During the Administration of Major General Norman T. Kirk." *Bulletin of the U.S. Army Medical Department* 7 (1947): 594–646.

Dougherty, Paul J., and Marlene DeMaio. "Major General Norman T. Kirk and Amputee Care During World War II." *Clinical Orthopaedics and Related Research*, Symposium: Recent Advances in Amputation Surgery and Rehabilitation, 472, no. 10 (June 6, 2014): 3107–13. https://doi.org/10.1007/s1199901436796.

Downs Jr., Frederick. "Prosthetics in the VA: Past, Present, and Future." *U.S. Naval Institute Proceedings* 134, no. 2 (February 2008): 56–61.

Gallagher, John L. "Compression Therapy." *The American Journal of Nursing* 44, no. 5 (May 1944): 423–27.

Gaynes, Robert. "The Discovery of Penicillin: New Insights After More Than 75 Years of Clinical Use." *Emerging Infectious Diseases Journal* 23, no. 7 (May 2017): 849–53. https://doi.org/10.3201/eid2305.161556.

Grettler, David J. "Activity for Body and Mind: The Career of

Nora Staael Evert, Physical Therapy Pioneer." *South Dakota History* 47, no. 1 (Spring 2012): 66–92.

Harris, R. I. "Amputations." *The Journal of Bone and Joint Surgery* 26, no. 4 (October 1944): 626–34.

Hays, Marguerite. "Eugene F. Murphy, PhD and Early VA Research in Prosthetics and Sensory Aids." *Journal of Rehabilitation Research & Development*, JRRD Guest Editorial, 38, no. 2 (2001): viii.

Kirwan, William E. "Escape Tactics of German War Prisoners." *Journal of Criminal Law & Criminology* 35, no. 5 (February 1945): 357–66.

Licht, Sidney. "An Army General Hospital Medical Library." *Bulletin of the Medical Library Association* 32, no. 4 (October 1944): 456–66.

McAleer, James. "Mobility Redux: Post-World War II Prosthetics and Functional Aids for Veterans, 1945 to 2010." *Journal of Rehabilitation Research & Development*, JRRD Guest Editorial, 48, no. 2 (2011): vii–xvi. https://doi.org/10.1682.

Min, Kyungchan. "The History of Penicillin: A Successful Case of Government Intervention." *The Concord Review* 23, no. 1 (Fall 2012): 45–61.

Peterson, Leonard T. "The Army Amputation Program." *The Journal of Bone and Joint Surgery* 26, no. 4 (October 1944): 635–38.

Petry, Lucile. "U. S. Cadet Nurse Corps: Established under the Bolton Act." *The American Journal of Nursing* 43, no. 8 (August 1948): 704–8. https://doi.org/10.2307/3456272.

Pohl, Hans, and Stephanie Oak. "War & Military Mental Health: The U.S. Psychiatric Response in the 20th Century." *American Journal of Public Health* 97, no. 12 (n.d.): 2132–42.

"Proceedings of 33d National Convention of American Legion, 1951." *U.S. Congressional Serial Set* 11599 (1952): 269.

Rorke, M. A. "Music and the Wounded of World War II." *Journal of Music Therapy* 33, no. 3 (1996): 189–207.

Todd, Janice S., Jason P. Shurley, and Terry C. Todd. "Thomas L. DeLorme and the Science of Progressive Resistance Exercise." *The Journal of Strength & Conditioning Research* 26, no. 11 (November 2012): 2913–2923. https://doi.org/10.1519/JSC.0b013e31825adcb4.

Wilkinson, Ernest L. "The United States Court of Claims: Where Uncle Sam Is Always the Defendant." *American Bar Association Journal* 36 (February 1950): 89–92, 155–59.

Laws and Legal Cases

American Const. Co. v. United States, 123 Ct. Cl. 408 (United States Court of Claims 1952).

Temple, Tex. Land Conveyance, Pub. L. No. 90–197, 81 STAT. U.S. Code 582 (1967).

Letters

Bethea, James A. Typewritten. "Letter from James A. Bethea, Commanding General, McCloskey General Hospital, Temple, TX. to Helen Keller, New York, NY." Typewritten, November 27, 1944. American Foundation for the Blind. https://bit.ly/3aLgN2z.

Poage, W. R. "Letter from W. R. Poage to Hon. R. C. Tompkins," October 17, 1952. Olin E. Teague Veterans Administration Center Medical Library Archives.

Sebek, Dan A. "Veterans Administration Memorandum to Chief, Voluntary Service Re: Historical Information," November 9, 1981.

Magazine Articles

"First Case." *Time Magazine*, July 23, 1945.

"Flowers for the Road Back: Texas Rotarians Provide a Veterans Hospital with a Modern Greenhouse." *The Rotarian*, March 1947.

National Railway Historical Society., Lancaster Chapter, Inc.

"Trains of Mercy: World War II Hospital Trains."
Lancaster Dispatcher, September 2013.
"Prosthetics: Artificial Arms and Legs Repair the Handicaps of
Battle Wounds." *Life Magazine*, January 31, 1944.
Sliger, Thomas F. "48 Hours in Paradise." *The Rotarian*, January
1946.
Vernon, John. "Jim Crow, Meet Lieutenant Robinson: A 1944
Court-Martial." *Prologue Magazine*, Spring 2008.
https://www.archives.gov/publications/prologue/2008/
spring/robinson.html.

Miscellaneous Documents

Patison, Augustine. "The Story of Maggie McCloskey." Olin E.
Teague Veterans' Center, n.d.
Roosevelt, Franklin Delano, "Press Conference #762"
(Executive Offices of the President, August 19, 1941),
FDR Library, https://bit.ly/2S4pkqE.
Texas Historical Commission. "Prisoner of War Camps in
Texas." Texas Historical Commission, n.d.
https://www.thc.texas.gov/public/upload/texas-pow-
MS-lesson-plan.pdf.

Newspaper Articles

"$1,000 Donated to McCloskey Fund." *The Austin American-
Statesman*. December 27, 1944.
"3 Day Conference M'Closkey Hospital." *Corsicana Daily Sun*.
January 26, 1945.
"3 Troop Carrier Planes Bring 75 Patients to McCloskey." *The
Austin American-Statesman*. January 11, 1944.
"8 Girls in Pinafores Delight in Aide Work at McCloskey." *The
Austin American-Statesman*. May 21, 1944.
"11 Puppies Born to M'Closkey Mascot." *Unknown*. n.d.
"375 Soldiers, Ill or Wounded, Moved by Plane." *The Tyler
Morning Telegraph*. May 25, 1944.
"700 More Wounded Arrive at Temple." *The Austin American-*

Statesman. October 13, 1943.

"1000-Bed Capacity Planned by VA at McCloskey Unit." *The Waco News-Tribune*. February 5, 1947.

"A.A.U.W. Hears of Red Cross Work in County." *Belton Journal and Bell County Democrat*. November 12, 1942.

"Air Ambulances Filled Temple Skies in 1944." *Temple Daily Telegram*. January 7, 2019.

"Army Base Hospital Awarded Temple." *Temple Daily Telegram*. January 7, 1942.

"Army Gives Former Waco Surgeon Colonelcy." *The Austin American-Statesman*. December 13, 1944.

"Army Hospital Construction Will Start Early April." *Temple Daily Telegram*. March 15, 1942.

"Army Hospital Work Started." *Temple Daily Telegram*. March 8, 1942.

"Army Plans to Reduce Hospitals." *The Austin American-Statesman*. October 9, 1945.

"Army Seeks Better Limbs for Wounded." *Waxahachie Daily Light*. March 19, 1946.

"Army Will Close 18 More Hospitals." *New York Times*. January 11, 1946, TimesMachine edition.

"Austin Cadet Takes Last Phase of Training at Army Hospital." *The Austin American-Statesman*. June 18, 1944.

Barnard, William C. "Prisoners of War in Texas Rapidly Being Repatriated." *The Denton Record-Chronicle*, January 1, 1946.

"Battle-Scarred Heroes of Fighting 36th Tell of Grim Salerno Landing." *Paris News*. November 15, 1943.

Baukhage. "Washington Digest: Today's Battlefield Victims Get Speedy, Effective Care." *The Bartlett Tribune*. December 10, 1943.

Begeman, Jean. "Lord Halifax's Son, In Witty Speech to Legislature, Praises Texans Fighting in Europe." *The Austin American-Statesman*. March 16, 1945.

"Belton Red Cross Lagging in Making Surgical Dressings." *The Belton Journal and Bell County Democrat*. February 25, 1943.

Benoit, Patricia K. "Backroads: Air Ambulances Filled Temple Skies in 1944." *Temple Daily Telegram*. January 6, 2019. http://www.tdtnews.com/news/article_ecab8306-1209-11e9-937e-737040878d59.html.

———. "Backroads: Christmas Parade Is a Temple Tradition." *Temple Daily Telegram*. December 5, 2016. https://www.tdtnews.com/news/article_aaf866d2-bab2-11e6-a9cf-9b27125843dd.html.

———. "Backroads: Nursing a Need: Cadet Corps Filled Shortage in World War II." *Temple Daily Telegram*. March 11, 2019.

———. "Backroads: Penicillin Was Lifesaver to Soldiers During World War II." *Temple Daily Telegram*. May 27, 2019.

———. "Backroads: Railcars Used to Transport Troops to Temple Hospital." *Temple Daily Telegram*. July 24, 2016. http://www.tdtnews.com/news/article_d2b6a1fc-5216-11e6-b935-7f1335b58109.html.

———. "Backroads: Santa Fe Hospital: 'A Delightful Place to Be Ill.'" *Temple Daily Telegram*. January 6, 2014. http://www.tdtnews.com/news/article_93929454-769a-11e3-adbf-001a4bcf6878.html.

———. "Many Babies Born at McCloskey General Army Hospital." *Temple Daily Telegram*, December 28, 2011.

———. "Temple's Role in Saving Millions: Army Hospital One of First to Dispense Nation's 'Secret' Weapon." *Temple Daily Telegram*, August 24, 2010.

Blanding, Harry. "McCloskey Hospital One Building: Plant One of World's Largest." *Temple Daily Telegram*. November 4, 1942.

"Bobby Byrne's Skyliners Will Play at McCloskey." *The Austin American-Statesman*. June 26, 1944.

"Bond Rally and Auction Sale to Be Held Here Saturday." *Belton Journal and Bell County Democrat*. September 23, 1943.

"Broken in Body but Not in Spirit." *St. Cloud Times*. September 25, 1945.

Brooks, Raymond. "Cheery Spirit Dominant in Army Hospital." *The Austin American-Statesman*. August 18, 1944, sec.

Texas Topics.

———. "Former Head of 36th Sees His Wounded." *The Austin American-Statesman*. August 17, 1944.

"'Bundles for Britain' Drive Has Successful Opening Day." *Temple Daily Telegram*. February 4, 1941.

"Cadet Nurses Top Quota First Year." *The Courier-Journal*. July 1, 1944.

"Catholic Women Here Send Largest Cookie Jar to McCloskey." *The Cameron Herald*. March 1, 1945.

"Ceremony at McCloskey Honors Medical Department." *Belton Journal and Bell County Democrat*. July 26, 1945.

"Circus to Entertain McCloskey Wounded." *The Austin American-Statesman*. October 15, 1944.

"Civilian Personnel Office Handles All Non-Military Employment at McCloskey." *Temple Daily Telegram*. November 4, 1942.

"Clipping Bureau Furnishes McCloskey Hospital Veterans with Jokes and Cartoons." *The Austin American-Statesman*. January 14, 1945.

"Convalescing GIs Building Their Own Christmas At Army Hospital." *Lubbock Avalanche-Journal*. December 9, 1945.

Coppedge, Clay. "Lanky and the POWs." *Texas Escapes Online Magazine*, November 8, 2006, sec. Letters from Central Texas. http://www.texasescapes.com/ClayCoppedge/Lanky-and-the-POWs.htm.

———. "Temple Camp Housed German, Italian Prisoners." *Temple Daily Telegram*. May 20, 2007.

"County Survey Results Given." *Belton Journal and Bell County Democrat*. October 11, 1945.

"Court Rules Against U.S. in Claims Case." *The Daily Oklahoman*. October 8, 1952.

"Defense Saving Bond Campaign Started Here." *Temple Daily Telegram*. May 2, 1941.

Dietz, David. "Army Doctors." *The Pittsburgh Press*. April 22, 1944, sec. Science Today.

"Dispute Over Moving TB Patients Grows; Poage's Remark Hit." *Brownwood Bulletin*. October 17, 1952.

Easley, Tex. "VA Hospital Needs to Be Checked." *The Austin American-Statesman*. December 1, 1948.

"Employment Stays Steady at McCloskey." *Belton Journal and Bell County Democrat*. August 23, 1945.

"Familiar Landmark, Old City Standpipe Torn Down for Scrap." *Temple Daily Telegram*. July 10, 1941.

"Fatal Beating of War Prisoner at Hearne Eyed." *The Austin American-Statesman*. January 14, 1944.

"First Baby Born at McCloskey Honored on Birthday Tuesday." *Belton Journal and Bell County Democrat*. November 4, 1943.

"First Occupational Therapists Receive McClockey [sic] Diplomas." *Dallas Morning News*. June 24, 1945.

Fleming, Michael T. "United States Army Hospital Trains: A Brief History of American Rail Casualty Transportation." *Timetable: The Newsletter of the Piedmont Division, SER*. n.d.

"Floodlighted Ball Field in Temple Available for Central Texas Towns." *The Belton Journal and Bell County Democrat*. September 23, 1948.

"For Us, the Living." *The Rattler*. November 20, 1942.

"Former GI Keeps Word to Buddies." *The Indiana Gazette*. February 18, 1949.

"Fort Sam Houston Wins Softball Title." *The Shreveport Journal*. August 29, 1944.

"Four-C College Fall Term." *The Cameron Herald*. September 3, 1942.

"Garden Club Leaders Plan Beautification with McCloskey Head." *Southwestern Times*, January 18, 1945.

"Gehrig's Trophy Brings $1,000,000 in Bond Sales." *The Sporting News*, June 29, 1944.

"Gen. Bradley, V A Head, Makes Inspection Trip." *The Richland Beacon News*. April 27, 1946.

"Gordon P. Roman in Rome Invasion." *The Longview News Journal*. August 4, 1944.

Graham-Ashley, Heather. "Frank W. Mayborn Integral to Hood." *Fort Hood Sentinel*. March 7, 2013.

"Grave Shortage of Nurses in Army, Says Col. Zita Callaghan." *Belton Journal and Bell County Democrat*. December 28, 1944.

"Gray Ladies Ranks Thinned by Season." *The Belton Journal and Bell County Democrat*. July 26, 1945.

Gresham, Hill C. "Many Problems Facing Temple Need Solution." *Temple Daily Telegram*. January 25, 1942.

———. "Opening of Army Hospital Marks New Era in Growth of City of Temple." *Temple Daily Telegram*. November 4, 1942.

Hart, Weldon. "This Man Proves Both Arms Aren't Necessary." *The Austin American-Statesman*. September 13, 1945, sec. Your Capital City.

"Hearst Charge of Neglected Soldier Branded as False." *The Pittsburgh Press*. March 5, 1944.

"Here And There in Texas." *Lubbock Morning Avalanche*. November 12, 1943.

"Hero Tells Why Divorce Suit Filed." *The Austin American-Statesman*. August 1, 1945.

"High Percentage of Men Wounded in War Saved." *The Daily Times-News*. April 15, 1944.

"High-Ranking Officers with Fifth Army in Italy Arrive at McCloskey Hospital; Tell of Terrible Battles." *The Tyler Morning Telegraph*. April 25, 1944.

"Hitler Declares England Will Fall During New Year." *The Austin American-Statesman*. January 1, 1941.

"Holiday Travel Not Bad; Many Civilians Cooperating." *The Austin American-Statesman*. December 23, 1943.

"Hospital's Brig Is in Northeast Corner of Grounds." *Temple Daily Telegram*. November 4, 1942.

"Hospitals Bring Fame to Temple as Clinical, Surgical Center." *Temple Daily Telegram*. June 25, 1941.

"How Army Dentists Broke Nazi's Glass Eye Monopoly: Wounded Soldiers Faced Black Patches Until They Developed New Plastics." *The Milwaukee Journal*, April

26, 1945.

Humphrey, Walter R. "Army Cures Nerve Casualties." *The Monitor*. December 19, 1943.

———. "First Invasion Casualties Normandy Beaches Reach Hospital in Temple Tuesday." *Corsicana Daily Sun*. July 11, 1944.

———. "Thousands of Civilians Join in Army's Dedication of Hospital." *Temple Daily Telegram*. November 5, 1942.

———. "Wounded Don't Want Stares; Just A Chance to Get Along." *The Palm Beach Post*. June 10, 1945.

"Iron for Britain In Belton Grows." *Temple Daily Telegram*. May 1, 1941.

"It's a Cotton Christmas." *The Corpus Christi Caller-Times*. December 4, 1939.

"James E. Ferguson, Former Texas Governor, Dies at Austin Home." *Borger Daily Herald*. September 22, 1944.

"Jim McGoldrick Makes Trip with Magazines for McCloskey Vets." *Cameron Herald*. November 16, 1944.

"Johnson Urges Continued Work on Home Front." *The Austin American-Statesman*. December 23, 1943.

"Keep 'Em Flying Week Proclaimed by Mayor Mason." *Temple Daily Telegram*. August 19, 1941.

Kennedy, David M. "The Nation: On the Home Front; What Is Patriotism Without Sacrifice?" *The New York Times*, February 16, 2003, sec. Week in Review. https://www.nytimes.com/2003/02/16/weekinreview/the-nation-on-the-home-front-what-is-patriotism-without-sacrifice.html.

"Kindness, Happiness, Efficiency, Principles Underlying Treatment of Veterans at McCloskey General." *The Eagle*. July 19, 1945.

"Landscape Project Brings Contributions." *The Austin American-Statesman*. November 12, 1944.

"Legless Vets of Hospital in Texas Play Girl Cagers." *The Times*. February 28, 1946.

Levine, Susan. "In WWII, Patriotism Unified A Nation." *Washington Post*. May 23, 2004.

https://www.washingtonpost.com/archive/local/2004/ 05/23/in-wwii-patriotism-unified-a-nation/a605dcd6-f2da-42e0-ae00-83d990429aba/.

"Literary Contest Open to Patients at McCloskey." *The Austin American-Statesman*. October 9, 1944.

"Lost Battalion Texans at Temple." *The Monitor*. October 24, 1945.

"Lou Gehrig Trophy Auctioned Off at War Bond Fight." *The Big Spring Daily Herald*. June 21, 1944.

"Luther League Will Sponsor 'Cheer Fund': Money to Be Sent to McCloskey For Wounded Vets." *Rockdale Reporter and Messenger*. February 1, 1945.

"Maimed Veterans Invent Wheel-Chair Ball Game." *New York Times*. October 25, 1945.

"Major Gen. Kirk Visits McCloskey." *The Belton Journal and Bell County Democrat*, October 11, 1945.

"Malaria Principal Worry of Medics, McCloskey Shows." *The Waco Tribune-Herald*. October 17, 1943.

"Mary Lela Engvall." *The Austin American-Statesman*. October 8, 1995, sec. Obituaries.

Mayborn, Frank W. "Temple Area Designated As 'Private Housing Priority Locality': New Quota Due." *Temple Daily Telegram*. April 14, 1942.

"McCloskey Hospital, Army's Largest, Observes First Anniversary." *Temple Daily Telegram*. November 4, 1943.

"McCloskey Hospital at Temple Has Nation's Largest Amputation Center." *The Marshall News Messenger*. May 7, 1944.

"McCloskey Hospital Dedication Nov. 4." *The Bartlett Tribune*, October 30, 1942.

"McCloskey Hospital Has Patients from Every Battlefront of This War." *El Paso Times*. May 21, 1944.

"McCloskey Hospital Put Back in Service." *The Austin American-Statesman*. April 4, 1946.

"McCloskey May Be Used in Veterans Hospital Set-Up." *The Austin American-Statesman*. January 24, 1946, sec.

Editorials.

"McCloskey Needs Nurses to Expand Services to Vets." *The Waco News-Tribune*. September 28, 1946.

"McCloskey Patient Marries at USO." *Belton Journal and Bell County Democrat*. August 2, 1945.

"McCloskey Patients Get $206.75 From Local Benefit Dance." *The West News*, n.d.

"McCloskey Purple Hearters One-Legged Court Wizards." *The Tennessean*. February 28, 1946.

"McCloskey Receives First Cadet Nurses." *Pampa Daily News*. June 23, 1944, sec. Back the Fifth.

"McCloskey Reconditions Vets for Civilian Life." *Denton Record-Chronicle*. July 13, 1945, sec. Texas Today.

"McCloskey Soldier-Patients Appointed Hospital Guides." *The Austin American-Statesman*. May 21, 1944.

"McCloskey Soldiers Start Move into New Barracks This Week; Library Equipped, Open; Bethea Has Army Anniversary: 92nd's C.O. Now Colonel." *Temple Daily Telegram*. n.d.

"McCloskey VA Center Cited for Efficiency." *The Waco Tribune-Herald*. October 2, 1960.

"McCloskey Vets Entertained by Westwood Country Club: Warm Hospitality Means Much to Crippled Soldiers." *Southwestern Times*, December 14, 1944.

"McCloskey Vets Push 5th Loan." *The Austin American-Statesman*. August 11, 1944.

McCullam, William. "Hands Gone, Blind, Deaf, Boy Left to Shift for Himself by Army." *San Francisco Examiner*. January 25, 1944.

"M'Closkey Gets Navarro County Champion Steer." *Corsicana Semi-Weekly Light*. October 3, 1944.

"Men from Nazi Camps Arrive at McCloskey." *Abilene Reporter-News*. March 5, 1945.

"Michro-Filmed Books Available for Hospitals." *Belton Journal and Bell County Democrat*. January 21, 1946.

"Miss Phillips Is Therapist Aid at McCloskey General Hospital." *The Belton Journal and Bell County Democrat*. April 5, 1945.

Mouche, Carol. "Area Residents Recall Temple's Prisoner-of-War Camp." *Temple Daily Telegram*. May 5, 1985.

"New Magic Metal Working Miracles for War Wounded." *Lubbock Morning Avalanche*. February 8, 1944.

"New School Radio Series Opens Today." *Temple Daily Telegram*. February 4, 1941.

"New U.S. Production Peak Is Due In 1941." *Temple Daily Telegram*. January 1, 1941.

"News of Men and Women in Uniform." *Belton Journal and Bell County Democrat*. February 7, 1946.

"No Limbs Needed in This Baseball Loop." *El Paso Times*. October 28, 1945.

"Officials at McCloskey Cancel Minstrel Show." *Taylor Daily Press*. April 8, 1945.

Olsen, Homer G. "Food Is Good and Plentiful at McCloskey General Hospital." *The Austin American-Statesman*. March 13, 1944.

———. "Former Hearst Writer Upholds Officers of Hospital Staff." *The Pittsburgh Press*. March 5, 1944.

———. "McCloskey Men Rebuild Own Health, Morale: Occupational Therapy Division Stresses Work by Hand." *The Austin American-Statesman*. March 10, 1944.

———. "Sick Returned to Active Life at McCloskey." *The Austin American-Statesman*. March 8, 1944.

———. "Teamwork Counts, McCloskey Medical Officer Says, Where Patient Comes First." *The Austin American-Statesman*. March 9, 1944.

"One Legged Vet Wins Jitterbug Contest." *The Austin American-Statesman*. January 23, 1946.

"One Thing Is Sure--Soldier Patients Won't Go Hungry." *Temple Daily Telegram*. November 4, 1942.

"One-Legged Vets Play Gal Cagers." *The Montana Standard*. February 28, 1946.

"Parts of World War 1 Plane Added to Aluminum Pile Here." *Temple Daily Telegram*. July 25, 1941.

Patrick, William C. "Army, Navy Doctors Report Big Gains in Saving Wounded." *The Salt Lake Tribune*. April 11, 1944.

Pearce, Dick. "Army Gives Refund to Disabled McCloud Vet."
  San Francisco Examiner. February 19, 1944.

"Penicillin at Hand." *Altoona Tribune*. December 14, 1943.

"Penicillin Drug Winning Fight to Save Life of Abilene Youth."
  Abilene Reporter-News. November 5, 1943.

"Penicillin Now in Mass Production." *The News*. December 14,
  1943.

"Penicillin on Way for Local Lad, Gravely Ill." *Abilene Reporter-
  News*. November 4, 1943.

"Penicillin Ready for Civilian Use." *Belton Journal and Bell
  County Democrat*. April 5, 1945.

"Penicillin Soon to Be Available in Ample Quantity." *The
  Morning Call*. December 14, 1943.

"Penicillin to Be Made Adequately Available." *Santa Cruz
  Sentinel*. December 15, 1943.

"Planes Take 254 Wounded." *The New York Times*. July 10,
  1944.

"Poems by McCloskey Men to Be Broadcast." *The Austin
  American-Statesman*. January 4, 1944.

"Pots and Pans Clatter Tune." *The Austin American-Statesman*.
  July 22, 1941.

Potter, Robert D. "Surgical Magic with Tantalum." *Pittsburgh
  Sun-Telegraph*. December 24, 1944.

"Principal Chief Nurse at Hospital Starting Her 25th Year of
  Service with Army." *Temple Daily Telegram*. November
  4, 1942.

"Pvt. WAAC Dog Veteran of Attu Fight at Hospital Here."
  Temple Daily Telegram. June 16, 1943.

"Red Cross Brings Xmas Cheer to Soldiers at McCloskey
  Hospital." *The Bartlett Tribune*, December 24, 1943.

"Red Cross Chapt. Begins Gray Lady Course October 9." *The
  Belton Journal and Bell County Democrat*. October 5,
  1944.

"Red Cross Still Has Many Calls for Its Services: Post-War Needs
  Keeps Bell County Chapter Very Busy." *The Belton
  Journal and Bell County Democrat*. December 19, 1946.

"Red Cross Work Is Praised by Mother of Wounded Man."

Belton Journal and Bell County Democrat. July 5, 1945.

"Rent Questionnaire Is Distributed Here." *Belton Journal and Bell County Democrat*. December 16, 1943.

"Request for Use of McCloskey By V A Awaits Action." *The Austin American-Statesman*. March 19, 1946, sec. Editorials.

"Requests for Penicillin." *The Evergreen Courant*. December 2, 1943, Town and Farm in Wartime edition.

"Returnee from Jap Prison Is Head Dietitian at McCloskey." *The Belton Journal and Bell County Democrat*. October 4, 1945.

"Rev. Thorn Will Head Belton Red Cross Campaign." *Belton Journal and Bell County Democrat*. February 25, 1943.

Russell, F. B. "Belton Needs Building Material." *Belton Journal and Bell County Democrat*. January 21, 1943.

"Salerno Veterans Guests of Nation." *Nebraska State Journal*. December 24, 1943.

"Shivers, Civic Leaders Battle Over Hospital." *El Paso Times*. October 10, 1952.

"Sick and Wounded Sing About Texas As Big Transport Wings Them to McCloskey Hospital." *Corsicana Semi-Weekly Light*. May 26, 1944.

"Skin and Bones Pictures Show True Prison Situation." *The Belton Journal and Bell County Democrat*. March 29, 1945.

"Slammin' Snead Exhibits Shots for McCloskey." *Abilene Reporter-News*. September 11, 1945.

"Soldiers in Texas Army Hospitals Have Good Christmas With Home Only in Their Dreams." *The Austin American-Statesman*. December 26, 1943.

"Solon Proposes to Name McCloskey for 36th Division." *Waco News-Tribune*. March 21, 1947.

Stimpson, George. "Capital Comment." *The Big Spring Daily Herald*. January 11, 1944.

"Temple Fight to End with VA Decision." *The Waco News-Tribune*. October 11, 1952.

"Temple Given Multi-Million War Hospital." *The Clifton Record*.

January 16, 1942.

"Temple Junior College Obtains New Property." *Waco Tribune Herald*. April 6, 1968.

"Temple Resolutions Oppose TB Patients in McCloskey." *The Waco News-Tribune*. October 8, 1952.

"Temple VA Center Hospital Dedication Section." *Temple Daily Telegram*. June 17, 1967, VA Hospital Dedication Edition.

"Temple Veterans Hospital May Get Increase in Beds." *Lubbock Morning Avalanche*. April 29, 1948.

"Temple's March of Pans Gets Splendid Start." *Temple Daily Telegram*. July 22, 1941.

"Texas Farm News." *Belton Journal and Bell County Democrat*. May 20, 1943.

"Texas Hospital Heals Wounded from War Areas." *Valley Evening Monitor*. November 11, 1943.

"Texas Inland Fishing Outlook Good as Summer Moves In." *Abilene Reporter-News*. May 25, 1945.

"The Facts About John Lindsey's Baseball Wound." *The Big Spring Daily Herald*. March 6, 1945.

""The Going Is Hard, But the Fight Is Well Worth It, Major McCloskey Wrote in Last Letter Before He Was Killed." *Temple Daily Telegram*. November 4, 1942.

"The Texan's Share in Winning World War 2." *The Denison Press*. September 8, 1944.

"They Still Know How to Shoot." *The Austin American-Statesman*. January 3, 1945.

Thompson, Fred D. "Wounded War Heroes from McCloskey To Help Austin Launch Bond Campaign." *The Austin American-Statesman*. January 11, 1944.

"Three Special Trains Weekly Bring Wounded Service Men to McCloskey, Largest Army Hospital in Nation." *The Eagle*. November 9, 1943.

"Three-Ton Load of Aluminum Sent from Bell County." *Temple Daily Telegram*. August 3, 1941.

"To Boys at McCloskey." *The Austin American-Statesman*. December 23, 1943, sec. Town Talk.

"Trees Sent to Hospital by Women." *The Austin American-Statesman*. January 23, 1955.

"T.S.C.W. New "Musical Charm: Program to Make Debut Saturday and Sunday at McCloskey Army Hospital." *Denton Record-Chronicle*. November 9, 1944.

"U.S. Army Camp Will Be Built at Killeen." *Belton Journal and Bell County Democrat*. January 15, 1942.

"VA Hospital in Temple to Stage State Golf Meet." *Waco News-Tribune*. August 10, 1946.

"Veterans Protest Plan to Abandon McCloskey." *The Cameron Herald and Centinel*. November 28, 1946.

"War Wounded Make Many Practical Items." *Belton Journal and Bell County Democrat*. September 7, 1944.

"Warm Southwest Becomes Greatest Army Hospital and Convalescent Area." *Abilene Reporter-News*. April 9, 1944.

"Wife Already Knew Soldier Had Lost Leg." *The Austin American-Statesman*. April 10, 1944.

"Wounded from All Fronts Enter Huge Temple Army Hospital to Leave With Mended Bodies." *The Austin American-Statesman*. July 8, 1943.

"Wounded Soldiers Flown to Temple." *Denton Record-Chronicle*. January 11, 1944.

Reports

"Annual Report of the Surgeon General. United States Army. Fiscal Year...," 1942. https://history.amedd.army.mil/booksdocs/Annual_Reports/1942_AHR.pdf.

Bethea, James A. "Annual Report of McCloskey General Hospital, Temple, Texas For the Calendar Year 1944." Temple, TX: McCloskey General Hospital, January 1, 1945.

———. "Annual Report of McCloskey General Hospital, Temple, Texas For the Calendar Year 1945." Temple, TX: McCloskey General Hospital, January 1, 1946.

Hannah, Lindsay. "United States Third Generation Veterans Hospitals, 1946-1958." Washington, DC: National Park Service, Winter 2017. https://www.dot7.state.pa.us/CRGIS_Attachments/Survey/2018M001042A_01H.pdf.

Kamarck, Kristy N. "The Selective Service System and Draft Registration: Issues for Congress." CRS Report. Washington, DC: Congressional Research Service, January 28, 2019. https://crsreports.congress.gov/product/pdf/R/R44452.

Kirk, Norman T. "Memorandum for Control Division, Services of Supply." Annual report. Surgeon General of the United States Army, August 18, 1942.

Marble, Sanders. "Rehabilitating the Wounded: Historical Perspective on Army Policy." Research. Falls Church, VA: Office of Medical History, Office of the Surgeon General, July 2008.

Theses and Dissertations

Baptiste, Joseph C. "The Enemy Among Us: World War II Prisoners of War." Dissertation, Texas Christian University, 1976.

Gregory, Kurt. "The German World War Two Prisoner and His Experience in the United States." Master's, California State University, 2001.

Hughes, Clifford Joseph. "A Study of Temple, Texas During World War II." Master's, Southwest Texas State University, 1972.

Landry, Meghann Lanae. "Fashioning the Future: The U.S. Cadet Nurse Corps, 1943-1948." Master's, Louisiana State University, 2012.

Loughlin, Richard Lawrence. "An Historical Study of Convalescent Reconditioning and Rehabilitation in the United States Army Hospitals." Ph.D., New York University, 1947.

Pearson, Alec Philmore, Jr. "Olin E. Teague and the Veterans' Administration." Texas A&M University, 1977.

Pluth, Edward John. "The Administration and Operation of German Prisoner of War Camps in the United States During World War II." Ph.D., Ball State University, 1970. ProQuest Dissertations & Theses Global.

Walker, Richard Paul. "Prisoners of War in Texas During World War II." Dissertation, North Texas State University, 1980.

Video

Army Service Forces. *Meet McGonegal, 1944*. 16 mm. Vol. Misc. 956. 2 reels vols. Official Film, War Department. Washington, DC, 1944. https://www.youtube.com/watch?v=FSLj5_HgYlo

Web Pages

Wiley G. Clarkson, Fort Worth Architect. "A History of His Architecture." Accessed January 23, 2019. http://www.clarksons.org/Clarkson/temple.htm.

United States Holocaust Memorial Museum. "Americans and the Holocaust." Accessed February 29, 2020. https://exhibitions.ushmm.org/americans-and-the-holocaust/us-public-opinion-world-war-II-1939-1941.

Ammentorp, Steen. "Bethea, James Albertus." Generals of World War II, c2000. http://www.generals.dk/.

City of Temple. "Draughon-Miller Central Texas Regional Airport | Temple, TX." Accessed March 7, 2020. https://www.ci.temple.tx.us/88/Airport-Services.

Gillespie, Robert S. "Army Hospital Trains." Railway Surgery, 2006. http://railwaysurgery.org/Army.htm.

Bell County Medical Alliance. "History of Bell County Medical Alliance," January 2015. http://www.bellcountymedicalalliance.com/history.html.

Texas Board of Nursing. "History- Texas Board of Nursing,"

2013. https://www.bon.texas.gov/history.asp.

LeBlanc, Robyn. "Foy Roberson." Memorials in Stone, 2018. http://ochceng105.web.unc.edu/biographies/foy-roberson/.

Findagrave. "MG James Albertus Bethea (1887-1984) - Find A..." Accessed January 23, 2019. https://www.findagrave.com/memorial/363564/james-albertus-bethea.

City of Temple. "Old Nine Temple College Golf Course 2600 South 1st Street," n.d. https://www.ci.temple.tx.us/DocumentCenter/View/12769/Old-Nine-Temple-College-Golf-Course?bidId=.

Peters, Gerhard, and John T. Woolley. "Proclamation 2352— Proclaiming a National Emergency in Connection with the Observance, Safeguarding, and Enforcement of Neutrality and the Strengthening of the National Defense Within the Limits of Peace-Time Authorizations." The American Presidency Project. Accessed February 18, 2019. https://www.presidency.ucsb.edu/node/210003.

Roosevelt, Franklin Delano. "May 27, 1941: Fireside Chat 17: On an Unlimited National Emergency." University of Virginia. Miller Center, May 27, 1941. https://millercenter.org/the-presidency/presidential-speeches/may-27-1941-fireside-chat-17-unlimited-national-emergency.

Ryan, Terri Jo. "Brazos Past: Waco's 4C Business School Opened Doors 90 Years Ago." WacoTrib.com. Accessed December 2, 2019. https://www.wacotrib.com/news/local/brazos-past-waco-s-c-business-school-opened-doors-years/article_7daa4f57-428e-52e5-9a1b-cd79374f5133.html.

Texas A&M College of Architecture. "F.W. Hensel." Outstanding Alumni, 2019. https://www.arch.tamu.edu/community/formerstudents/outstanding-alumni/past-honorees/32/.

Truman, Harry S. "Rear Platform and Other Informal Remarks in Texas | Harry S. Truman." Truman Library, September 27, 1948. https://www.trumanlibrary.gov/library/public-papers/212/rear-platform-and-other-informal-remarks-texas.

"Victory Parade of Spotlight Bands | Variety | Old Time Radio Downloads." Accessed July 8, 2019. https://www.oldtimeradiodownloads.com/variety/victory-parade-of-spotlight-bands/4.

The American Red Cross. "World War II and the American Red Cross," n.d. https://www.redcross.org/content/dam/redcross/National/history-wwii.pdf.

Index of Personal Names

Now to Him who is able to keep you from stumbling, and to make you stand in the presence of His glory blameless with great joy, to the only God our Savior, through Jesus Christ our Lord, be glory, majesty, dominion and authority, before all time and now and forever. Amen. ~Jude 24-25